What Readers Are Saying About Books from Robert Lesslie. MD

~~~~

Notes from a Doctor's Pocket

"I just finished reading *Notes from a Doctor's Pocket* and am thrilled to know that you'll have another book out this fall…All your books have been enjoyed by our household…keep it up!"

Brenda

"I've never enjoyed anything as much as your books in a long time…I live by myself and found myself laughing, crying, etc. My dog wondered, 'What in the world?'!"

Connie

"Besides the combination of page-turning inspirational adventure, I and my family want to thank you for providing a window into the world of emergent medicine without the coarseness, profanity, and unnecessary sexual content one usually finds in this genre…May God continue to richly bless your work!"

Howard

Angels on the Night Shift

"A very moving, yet compassionate, story of a caring doctor's life."

Wes

"Fast-paced, fascinating, well-written, and absorbing…I thoroughly enjoyed this and will certainly be looking out for any other books written by this medical author."

TheGardenWindow.blogspot.com

"I love your books! Always wondering who will burst through those doors next! Some of the stories are heartbreaking, some are encouraging, but all of them motivate me to become the best nurse possible. I can't wait for the next one!"

Ruth

Angels and Heroes

"When I started I could not put this book down…It made me realize that there are still good people on earth. I am a full-time police officer and a volunteer firefighter/EMS. I can't wait to pass this book on to others in my field."

Gary

"What stories are held in this book—people wh~ ʲuˢᵗ ᵍo the whole way to be a help and sacrifice their lives! I am not much of a r⸺ ⸺⸺⸺ but I fell in love with this book."

"I worked 14 years at a hospital in various positions—the last was in the CCU as a monitor tech and secretary. I honestly felt like I was working alongside you and all the staff mentioned in your books!…I tried not to read too fast because I didn't want the books to end!"

Louise

Angels on Call

"As an assistant principal…I have reflected on my own life's work with adolescent students as I read each account…I am writing to share how very much I enjoyed your book, especially the inspiring scriptural references accompanying each story."

Don

"Thank you for the two *amazingly awesome* books you have written. As a Christian pursuing a career in medicine, I find them really inspiring. I had tears in my eyes many times, especially in *Angels on Call.* I love, love, love these books!"

Alina

"The book was an inspiration during a difficult time in our lives…Your humility and humanity jumped out at me. I truly believe God works through us and that there are angels among us."

Chuck

Angels in the ER

"With 5 children and 17 grandchildren, I have spent many stressful times in various ERs, and too often we do not see that we parents, grandparents, or patients are not the only ones stressed out. The hospital staff has decisions to make, families to comfort, and unruly people to deal with. *Thank you and your fellow workers for all you do…* and keep the books coming!"

Vicki

"My father died in the ER and this is what drew me to your book *Angels in the ER.* I was searching for something spiritual in nature and your title grabbed my eye. So there you go—God had a plan and I found your wonderful book…We wish you all the very best."

Vic

"The most inspiring and relatable book I have read throughout my college career in nursing school…I often feel that my small contributions of extra time with patients or a simple smile have no impact on anyone's life. I was inspired by your book and appreciated the Bible verses throughout."

Katie

"I am a busy working mother but managed to read the entire book in less than three days. The way you described the people and the situations was brilliant…You see things in a very special way and have made me see…thank you."

Jamie

MIRACLES
in the ER

Robert D. Lesslie, MD

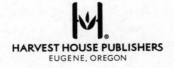

HARVEST HOUSE PUBLISHERS
EUGENE, OREGON

Cover by Left Coast Design, Portland, Oregon

Cover photo © bikeriderlondon / Shutterstock

All the incidents described in this book are true. Where individuals may be identifiable, they have granted the author and the publisher the right to use their names, stories, and/or facts of their lives in all manners, including composite or altered representations. In all other cases, names, circumstances, descriptions, and details have been changed to render individuals unidentifiable.

MIRACLES IN THE ER
Copyright © 2014 by Robert D. Lesslie, MD
Published by Harvest House Publishers
Eugene, Oregon 97402
www.harvesthousepublishers.com

Library of Congress Cataloging-in-Publication Data
Lesslie, Robert D., 1951-
Miracles in the ER / Robert D. Lesslie, MD.
    pages cm
ISBN 978-0-7369-5482-2 (pbk.)
ISBN 978-0-7369-5484-6 (eBook)
1. Hospitals—Emergency services—Popular works. 2. Emergency medical personnel—Popular works. 3. Medical emergencies—Popular works. I. Title. II Title: Miracles in the emergency room.
RA975.5.E5L48 2014
616.02'5092—dc23

                                                          2014002581

Printed in the United States of America

        15 16 17 18 19 20 21 22 / BP-CD / 10 9 8 7 6 5 4

To Barbara—my wife and editor in chief

And to my grandchildren,
the surest evidence of miracles in my life—
Jack Sullivan
Connor Thomas
Denton Lesslie
Caris Ann
Christian Nathaniel
Adah Elizabeth
…and those to come

Contents

Layout of the ER

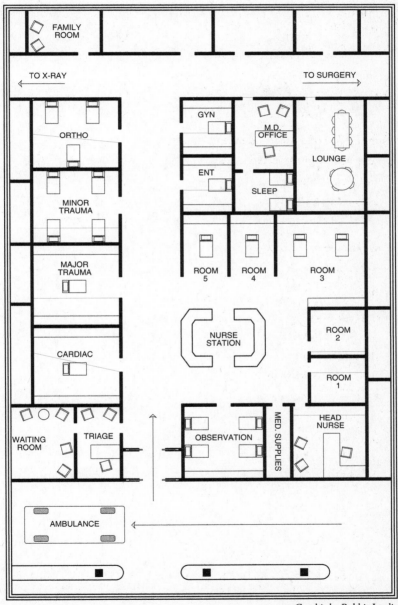

Graphic by Robbie Lesslie

D oc, I'm tellin' ya, it was a miracle!"
        Fresh out of my residency, when one of our ER patients would tell me this, my usual response was to assume the "position"—one arm folded across my chest, my chin cupped in the other hand. Slowly nodding my head, I would patiently wait until he—or she—finished, then get on with the matter at hand.

Not that my faith didn't allow for the occurrence of miracles, or unexpected acts of God. It was just that the ER didn't seem a likely place for these things to happen.

That was more than thirty years ago, and things have changed. Or at least I have changed. The "position" now is to pull up a stool, rub my hands together, and say, "Tell me about it." I have seen and experienced too many unexplainable things to discount anyone's story and the ability and willingness of the Lord to act directly in our lives.

As it turns out, the ER is just the place for miracles. We deal with matters of life and death, joy and grief, happiness and sorrow. And we deal with people from all walks of life and with every imaginable—sometimes *unimaginable*—problem. Why shouldn't we expect to find the Lord in this place? And if things happen that we can't explain, whose shortcoming is that? If we open our eyes and our hearts, we soon come to agree with C.S. Lewis when he wrote,

> *Miracles do not, in fact,*
> *break the laws of nature.*

To the contrary, it seems that miracles are a natural and intentional part of creation—and a very real part of each of our lives. If only we had eyes to see.

Days pass, years vanish
and we walk sightless among miracles.

ATTRIBUTED TO A JEWISH SABBATH PRAYER

THE *Miracle* OF HEALING

And Jesus said to him,
"What do you want me to do for you?"
And the blind man said,
"Rabbi, let me recover my sight."
And Jesus said to him,
"Go your way;
your faith has made you well."
And immediately he recovered his sight
and followed him on the way.

MARK 10:51-52 ESV

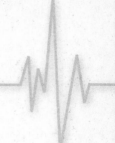

Let It Be

The helicopter blades thumped in the dark, cold night—barely seventy-five yards from the closed ambulance-entrance doors. Ricky Adler was being flown to the trauma center in Charlotte and to a waiting neurosurgeon.

Ricky was lucky. He had been working the graveyard shift at a local manufacturing company and had fallen twenty feet from a platform. His right wrist had been fractured, but more significantly, so had his neck. EMS 1 brought him to the ER, where we stabilized him and arranged for his transfer.

The collective adrenaline rush was subsiding, and several of us were standing and sitting around the nurses' station.

The thumping outside slowly faded into a welcomed silence, all too soon broken by Joel Carver, the young paramedic from EMS 1. "I don't know how he survived that fall, Doc. Twenty feet is a long way."

"He was moving everything—his arms and legs," Carla ventured. "That's a good sign, don't you think?" She was one of our third-shift nurses and had been in major trauma with Adler.

"Yeah," I agreed. "That's a good sign. And I agree with you, Joel. Falling twenty feet and surviving is—"

"It's a miracle." Amy Connors finished my sentence. "Gotta be a miracle."

Joel shook his head and looked over at me. "Doc, when was the last time you saw a *real* miracle—something you couldn't explain?"

I was sitting in a chair behind the desk and rolled it back, stretching out my legs. I was tired.

"Joel, I would say what we just saw with Ricky Adler is something that's hard to explain. I showed you his X-rays, didn't I? He has two fractures in his neck and the C-3 vertebra is riding *way* over C-4. And yet he doesn't have any spinal-cord injury. Like Carla said, he's moving everything.

17

When they get him to the OR and get that fracture stabilized, he'll be fine. He might end up having more trouble from his wrist than his neck. Explain that one." I raised my eyebrows and looked at the paramedic.

"I hear ya, Doc." Joel was standing on the other side of the counter, his forearms resting on its surface. "But you know what I mean. People talk about miracles and strange things happening—brain tumors disappearing and people regaining their vision after fifty years. When's the last time you saw anything like that?"

I closed my eyes, folded my hands behind my head, and searched my fatigued memory banks.

And there, filed safely away, was the image of three-year-old Bobby McManus lying unconscious on the stretcher in major trauma.

———

Gerald McManus was in the backyard, throwing a baseball with his oldest son, Andy. The twelve-year-old had a promising arm and Gerald was giving him pointers on how to throw a slider.

The ball thwacked into Gerald's webbed glove. "That's better, Andy. *Now* you're starting to get some action on it."

The boy grinned and slapped the leather of his oversized outfielder's mitt. "Come on, Dad, bring the heat!"

Gerald hesitated and cocked his head. "You sure about that?"

"Bring it, Dad!" Andy taunted.

Gerald went into his pitcher's windup, checked an invisible first base, glanced over his right shoulder at a nonexistent runner on third, looked up at the cloudless sky, and let fly.

He didn't see Bobby bolt around the garage and head straight for Andy.

The sound—a loud *thud*—was sickening, and would forever haunt Gerald's dreams.

The three-year-old crumpled to the ground as if he were a deer shot from a tree stand.

"Bobby!" Gerald screamed. He ripped off his glove and threw it onto the grass. "Bobby!"

He cradled the unconscious child in his arms and looked up at Andy. "Go get your mother! Tell her to call 9-1-1!"

Andy stood frozen, his eyes wide and mouth open. Every bit of color drained from his face and his legs trembled. He didn't move.

"Go!"

This time he took a few hesitant steps toward the house, then burst into a sprint. With head back and elbows flying, he yelled, "Momma!" over and over again.

"What do you make of this?" Drew Pritchard asked. The young ER physician was pointing to Bobby McManus's pupils. They were both larger than normal and deviated to his right side. That's where the ball had struck his head, just behind the temporal area. His scalp was swollen and bruised, and I thought I could feel a step-off in the bones of his skull.

"He's bruised his brain," I answered, once again checking and not finding the boy's reflexes. "And he probably has a subdural. The eyes are supposed to look toward the side of the injury, so that makes sense."

"They're ready in CT." Amy stood in the doorway and stared at the small, motionless body on the stretcher. She shook her head, turned, and walked slowly back to the nurses' station. She had a son Bobby's age.

"Vital signs still stable," Lori told us. She stood at the head of the bed and was making notes on the clipboard for major trauma.

"Still doesn't react to pain, or verbal stimulation, or..." She was mumbling to herself, charting his neurologic status.

"Anything." I finished her sentence. "He doesn't respond to anything."

Drew and I talked with Bobby's parents while he was in CT. Gerald McManus sat on the edge of the small sofa in the family room, rubbing his hands together and staring at the floor.

"Is he better, Dr. Lesslie?" his wife asked.

"He's the same. Still not moving or responding, but he's breathing on his own...and that's good."

"Is he going to wake up?" she sobbed. "Is he going to be okay?"

Bobby did have a large right-sided subdural hematoma with evidence of significant bruising of the brain on that side of his head. And he didn't wake up.

We sent him by helicopter to Charlotte, where he would need an emergency operation. The hematoma would need to be drained and the pressure in his brain closely monitored. After that, it was a matter of time—watching and praying.

The surgery was a success, and the swelling in Bobby's brain gradually improved. He was moved from the neuro ICU to a less acute unit, where his family and friends could visit him more freely. His neurosurgeon was "cautiously optimistic," as Bobby's uncle would tell anyone who asked. But after three and a half weeks, the neurosurgeon was less "optimistic" and more "cautious." Bobby still did not respond or move—he remained in a coma.

"How long can this go on?" his mother repeatedly asked the surgeon. "When will he wake up?"

She didn't want the answer—not the *real* one. Bobby might never wake up, and the longer he remained like this—unresponsive, in a coma—the dimmer were his chances of a recovery.

A brain-wave study was inconclusive. "There's activity there," the parents were told. "But it's not normal. We'll just have to wait and see."

Wait and see. The three and a half weeks dragged into five, and then six.

But the McManuses were a strong family. Aunts and uncles and cousins visited and prayed and helped keep the vigil, never giving up hope—confident that one day Bobby would again be running through his backyard. And in spite of this unbearable stress, his mother and father hung together, supporting each other. Gerald was overcome—almost destroyed—by guilt, but his wife never wavered in her support of him. There was never a moment of blame or accusation. That was the only thread that kept Gerald from completely unraveling.

Seven weeks passed and Bobby remained the same—still in a coma, still unresponsive. That's when his great-grandfather, Virgil McManus, came to visit. Virgil was the ninety-seven-year-old patriarch of the family. Though his body had failed him years earlier, his mind was quick and agile. He resided in a retirement center and couldn't travel. But on this day he demanded that he be taken to the hospital to see his great-grandson.

Virgil's wheelchair was rolled into the boy's room and over to Bobby's bed. For a long, silent moment, he looked down on the motionless body lying under a single thin sheet.

Slowly, Virgil's weak and trembling hand stretched over the boy and gently came to rest on his forehead. The old man closed his eyes and his head dropped to his chest.

"Lord, if it's your will that Bobby recover and wake up—let it be."

Joel's eyes were locked on mine. I leaned back in my chair, exhausted by the memory and retelling of this story.

"What happened, Doc? Tell me." The paramedic edged closer.

I took a deep breath and sighed. This part was always difficult for me.

"Two days later, Bobby woke up. It was gradual, but within another day or so he was talking and walking and ready to go home. He didn't remember anything that had happened—not the baseball or the hospital or his great-grandfather's visit. Still doesn't. But he's completely normal and doing fine."

Joel nodded slowly and looked down at the floor.

A quiet moment passed. He looked up at me and said, "That's an amazing story. But Doc, I gotta ask ya. How do you know it's true? Were you there with his great-grandfather? When Bobby woke up?"

"I *know* it's true. I've seen him, and now he's a completely normal six-year-old. But no, I wasn't there."

I motioned with my head to the cardiac room, where Carla was restocking supplies.

Joel turned and looked at the nurse.

"But *she* was," I said quietly. "That's Bobby's mother."

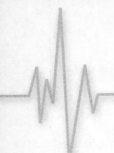

Gone

"Now, tell me again how this happened."

My hand rested on the teenager's ankle, carefully feeling for a pulse. It was still there, strong and bounding. Reassuring, considering the obvious fracture of his right femur.

EMS had just brought him in from one of the local high schools. He had been running the 440 in a track meet and had suddenly gone down with a little over a hundred yards to go.

One of the paramedics replied. "His coach said he heard a scream and looked just in time to see Ben grab his leg and fall to the ground." He had gone on to describe the obvious angulation of the boy's right thigh. He and his partner had immediately placed him in traction, started an IV, and brought him to the ER.

This still didn't make sense. Ben Stevens was a healthy, muscular four-teen-year-old with a fractured femur. There must have been something more to this injury—maybe a pothole in the track or an awkward plant of his foot with a sudden twisting of his leg. This kind of thing just didn't happen out of the clear blue.

"It was like I said, Doc. I was trying to pick up my speed, close strong, and then I felt a snap. Heard it too. And I went down."

We had given him something for the pain and he was lying comfort-ably on the trauma-room stretcher. His mother stood beside him, gently stroking his forehead, her own forehead furrowed. She was chewing one corner of her lip and didn't take her eyes off her boy.

The door to trauma burst open and a middle-aged man took two steps into the room, glanced around, then walked quickly over to the stretcher.

"Ben, are you alright?"

The man looked down at the boy, then over to his mother, and finally at me.

"Is he okay? What happened? Is he going to need surgery? What about—"

"It's okay, Dad—I'm going to be fine." Ben reached out a hand to his father. "Just a broken bone. Nothing serious."

John Stevens took his son's hand in both of his own and looked over at me again. "How did this happen? I thought he was at a track meet."

I told him what I knew, and Ben filled in the rest. While we were talking, two lab technicians came into the room and prepared to draw some blood. He would be going to the OR and we would need some basic lab work.

"Type and cross for four," I told them. A fractured femur can bleed a lot and he was going to need some blood.

Amy Connors stuck her head into the room. "They're ready for him in X-ray, and the orthopedist on call is on the way down."

Ben's femur was obviously fractured and I had made sure he didn't have tenderness anywhere else.

"Just the femur, right?" Amy called out again, raising her eyebrows at me.

"Yeah, that's all we need."

Ben coughed a couple of times and the rattling caused me to spin around.

"When did that start? The coughing?"

He looked up at me and shook his head. "I'm not sure. It's just a cough."

"I noticed it a couple of days ago." His mother stopped stroking his forehead and looked over at me. "Nothing bad, or anything. Just an occasional cough, mainly at night."

"Any chills or fever?" I looked at her and then at Ben.

He shook his head. "No, I've been fine."

I turned and faced Amy. "Let's get a chest X-ray too, PA and lateral."

"Got it." The door closed behind her and she was gone.

"Ben, have you had any broken bones before?"

"No, not that I can remember." He looked over at his mother, and she shook her head.

"How about your index finger?" His father interjected. "When you fell out of the tree house. Remember?"

"Oh yeah." Ben smiled and nodded his head. "That was nothing, just a little crack." He held up his left hand and pointed to the ceiling. "See. Fine."

"No medical problems or any medications?" I was still struggling to understand why this had happened.

"No, nothing like that." His mother put a finger to the side of her face. "We *did* take him to his pediatrician a month or so ago. He was having some leg pain." She paused and looked down at her son's splinted right leg. "I think it was this one, wasn't it?"

Ben put a hand on his injured thigh and nodded.

"He told us it was just 'growing pains,' and nothing to worry about."

"It was getting better, wasn't it, son?" His father leaned closer to the stretcher. "You haven't said anything about it lately."

Ben was silent, and his hand remained on his thigh. He took a deep breath and sighed.

"It was getting better, right?" his father repeated.

The door opened and two radiology techs walked into the room. "Ready to go to X-ray? This shouldn't take very long."

Twenty minutes later, the same two techs rolled Ben back into the trauma room. His labs had just been returned and I was studying them. He was a little anemic, but it looked chronic, not something that had happened this afternoon.

One of the techs snapped the X-ray of his femur onto the view box, then laid three or four other films on the counter. She glanced at me and when I looked in her direction, her gaze quickly shifted to the floor. She locked the wheels of Ben's stretcher and the two disappeared.

I was ten feet from the view box but could clearly see the mid-shaft fracture, angulated and shortened. It was what I expected.

As I walked closer, my heart flew into my throat and the blood drained from my face.

"What's the matter, Dr. Lesslie?" It was Ben's mother, and I didn't respond. I just stared at the X-ray. The femur was fractured, but the break was through bone that was irregular, haphazardly layered like…like onion rings. It was bone cancer, probably a sarcoma, and it looked aggressive and deadly.

The cough! I walked over to the view box, took down the X-ray of Ben's femur, and replaced it with the film of his chest.

I couldn't stifle a loud sigh, and his mother repeated, "Dr. Lesslie, *what* is the matter?"

I turned around and faced the three of them.

"Ben's femur is broken, just like we thought. But it broke through an area of what looks like bone cancer. And if it *is* cancer, it's already spread to his lungs."

I was with the family when the orthopedist confirmed my fears and explained what needed to be done. There would be no surgical repair of the fracture, no rodding of the broken femur. His leg was going to come off. And then there would be chemotherapy and maybe radiation. He was in a battle to save his life.

John Stevens stood beside his son's stretcher, head hanging down, silent. Ben's mother looked at the orthopedist and then at me, all the while gently patting her boy's shoulder.

"He's in the Lord's hands," she said quietly. "He's always been in the Lord's hands."

I saw Ben in the ER three months later. His parents brought him in with fever, chills, aches, and a persistent cough. He looked like he felt terrible—pale, sweating, shivering. Yet he managed a smile when he saw me.

"Hey, Doc. I'm not feelin' so good."

His parents filled me in on what had transpired since he fractured his leg. The amputation had gone well and he was already able to get around some, much better than any of his physicians—of which there were many—had thought possible.

"He's determined." His father nodded, looking down at Ben and smiling.

"He's hardheaded," Mrs. Stevens spoke up. "Just like his father."

Ben had lost some weight since that first visit. That was to be expected. I had talked with one of his oncologists shortly after the surgery about his outlook, and he had used the word "months" instead of "years." It was a bad cancer. There were the three aggressive tumors that I had seen in his lungs, and there was little hope that chemo would be able to stop them. Except for his chest, though, all of his other scans had been clear.

"We tried the chemotherapy," his mother explained when I asked about his treatment. "He just got so sick, and they stopped it after the second one. They haven't decided on what's next."

She grew quiet, and I focused on today's new problem. I was afraid he had pneumonia and that his lung cancers had spread.

"We'll need to get another chest X-ray and check that out. I want to be sure he doesn't have any infection there."

Ben's father looked sharply at me, then turned away.

"And since it's January, I'm going to get a flu test. We're seeing a lot of it now, and that might be a possibility."

No one said anything, and I walked to the door and called out to Amy, telling her what we needed.

Ben was rolled back into the department and over to room 4. His parents followed, along with one of the X-ray techs. She handed me his films, then helped him onto the stretcher.

I walked over to the view box, knowing what I was going to find and not wanting to look.

"Doc, the boy in 4 is positive for the flu. Type A."

I looked over at Amy Connors. She held a lab slip in her hand and waved it at me. That would explain the fever and aches and the cough. After all, even though he had metastatic bone cancer, he could still get the same things everyone else did. In fact, it was more likely. And the flu was no exception.

The X-ray of his chest snapped into place on the view box and I flipped on the bright light. I had to force myself to look up and—

His chest showed completely clear! There was no pneumonia and there was no cancer! I compared this X-ray with the one we had made three months earlier, carefully searching the areas where the tumors had been.

Gone! His lung cancers were gone! He just had the old-fashioned, run-of-the-mill flu!

I almost ran over to room 4, jerked the curtain aside, and told Ben and his parents the news.

Ben nodded and smiled calmly. His father stared at me, eyes wide and mouth open.

His mother gasped. Her hands flew to her mouth and tears flowed freely down her cheeks.

Gone.

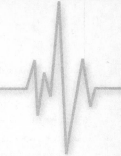

He Ain't Heavy…

"Still no pulse."

Jeff Ryan had his fingers on the man's left carotid artery. He glanced up at the clock on the wall. "It's been over forty minutes."

I looked at the cardiac monitor for the fiftieth time—flatline. Nothing.

Virginia Granger stepped into cardiac and walked up behind me. She put on a hand on my shoulder and said, "Time to call this one, Dr. Lesslie."

She was right, and I knew it.

"Okay, that's it." I glanced around the room at the nurses and techs surrounding the bed. "Thanks for your help."

"7:52 p.m.," Virginia announced. She made a note on Ted's chart and headed out of the room.

I stood at the head of the stretcher and watched as the staff slowly and quietly drifted through the doorway. One moment the room had been frenetic, charged with the energy of our efforts to save this man's life. And the next—it was as if the very walls uttered a whispered and final sigh.

He was only forty-two years old, and that made it even harder. I had seen him in the ER a couple of weeks earlier with a low-grade fever and what seemed like a simple virus. All of his labs had been okay, and there was nothing on his chest X-ray. He was a kidney-transplant patient, only six or seven months out from his surgery, and we needed to be especially careful with him. His family doctor had put him in the hospital for a few days and when everything had seemed fine, Ted Bartlett had been sent home.

Now he was on a stretcher in the cardiac room—dead. His lab work looked as if his kidneys had suddenly shut down, and he had an overwhelming infection due to the immune system suppressants he was taking. That was the probable explanation for his death, but it didn't make anything easier.

Lori Davidson cleared her throat and I looked over at her. We were alone in the room.

"I'll take care of things and see if he has any family members in the waiting room." She didn't look up from the pile of papers and rhythm strips scattered on the countertop.

Virginia was standing at the nurses' station and I walked up beside her.

"His mother and I were good friends—*are* good friends," she corrected herself. "She developed dementia a couple of years ago and it's gotten a lot worse lately. She's in a long-term care facility now and isn't able to communicate."

I nodded in the direction of the cardiac room. "Does he have any other family in town or nearby?"

"Just *that* man." Virginia was looking over my shoulder and I twisted around. "His brother."

Lori was leading a slender, middle-aged man down the hallway and into cardiac.

"Good. I'll go—"

"Hold on just a second." The head nurse laid her hand on my forearm, and I turned to face her. "There are a few things you need to know about Andrew Bartlett."

Andrew was four years younger than his brother and had always walked in Ted's shadow, or at least he thought so. Ted was a three-letter athlete at the local high school and had won the state track championship in the half-mile. Everything seemed to come easy for Ted—sports, friends, girls, studies. It was just the opposite for Andrew. He tried out for the football team but didn't make the first cut. The coaches voiced their surprise and disappointment, given the successes of his older brother.

None of this was lost on the younger boy. His frustration turned to resentment toward his brother and ultimately to anger. Ted didn't understand it and didn't know how to deal with the animosity. His years in college created more space between the two brothers—a distance that grew and was never bridged.

Years passed. Then Ted became sick. Out of nowhere, his kidneys stopped working. The specialists had no clue and no answers. Multiple biopsies weren't helpful and no treatments could stave off the inevitable. He was soon on dialysis, every other day. And then every day. Even that was only temporizing. The only hope for Ted Bartlett was a kidney transplant.

The doctors turned first to any family members who might be a good match. His mother was quickly ruled out, and Ted's father had died years earlier in an auto accident. That left Andrew, and he would have nothing to do with it. He said he was too busy, too much going on, and he couldn't take the chance of getting sick.

Because of Ted's age and previous good health, he was high up on the transplant list. But there were no good matches and without that, the chances were too great that an operation would fail. All the while he was getting sicker and weaker.

"It was finally his mother who talked some sense into Andrew." Virginia shook her head and stared at the countertop. "To this day I don't know what she told that boy, but something changed his mind. He lived in Charleston, so it wasn't much of a trip to get here. When they tested him, he was a perfect match. I remember talking to one of the doctors, and he was amazed at how good it was. He thought they must have been identical twins." She shook her head again and chuckled. "Far from that."

The surgery had gone well, and both brothers quickly recovered. Ted was soon doing fine, off his dialysis, and only taking a couple of medications to keep his body from rejecting his brother's kidney. Andrew was back in Charleston.

"That's good to know, Ms. Granger." I nodded at the nurse and was turning around when I felt her hand on my arm again.

"That's not all, Dr. Lesslie." Her voice was quiet, strained, and I faced her once again.

"A few weeks after the procedure, Andrew was getting some routine follow-up labs and his white count was elevated. Not bad, but enough to cause the doctors to repeat the study in a week. The *second* time it was sky-high—over 30,000—and within a few days he was diagnosed with acute leukemia. Funny how things work sometimes. He wasn't one to go to the doctor very often, if at all. If Ted hadn't needed a transplant and if Andrew... Anyway, he got sick real fast. You can guess what happened next."

I shook my head and said, "He needed a bone-marrow transplant, and the best donor was going to be his brother, Ted."

"The *only* donor," Virginia said. "No other matches came close. They were only a few months out from the kidney transplant and the doctors were reluctant to consider it. But Andrew was getting sicker, and Ted insisted."

"You'd think with all the medications there might be some problems." I rubbed my chin, trying to get my head around all this.

"That's why the doctors were reluctant to do it. But Ted was insistent and determined. His brother had saved his life and now he had a chance to do the same for him. But you know, it worked. Ted never missed a beat—no setbacks or anything. And the bone-marrow transport was a complete take. As far as I know, Andrew's been in remission ever since."

"Wow, that's some story." I watched Virginia's eyes, waiting. Was there something more she needed to tell me?

"Anything else?"

She sighed and pressed her starched, white uniform with the palms of her hands. Then she looked at me over her bifocals. "That's not enough?"

The door to cardiac opened and Lori stepped into the hallway. Our eyes met, she nodded, then turned and walked away.

Andrew Bartlett was standing at the side of the stretcher, leaning over his brother and holding Ted's hands in both of his own. I walked over and he looked up.

"You're Dr. Lesslie?"

I nodded.

"Thanks for trying to help Ted. The nurse told me you worked with him a long time and that..." His voice broke and he turned away.

"We did everything we could. There was just too much going against him."

We didn't say anything for a moment.

"It was his time, I guess." Andrew spoke quietly. "At least that's what Momma would say. And she would probably be right."

We were silent again, and then he looked up at me.

"The last couple of months, Ted and I talked a lot. It was just last week that he said..." His voice was breaking again but he cleared his throat and struggled to continue. "He said that his kidney failure was a gift—a miracle. If he hadn't needed a transplant and if I hadn't been the donor and had the follow-up blood work—who knows what would have happened? It might be *me* lying on this stretcher."

Andrew looked down at the peaceful face of his brother, took a deep breath, and sighed.

"He said we should make the most of this. It was a chance for us to live our lives like we meant it, and to always remember it can be over in the blink of an eye. He said his kidney failure and my leukemia were a miracle. He said they were a gift."

...he's my brother.

Sometimes, You Just Know

Early October, and the weather had finally changed. The summer had been long and hot, but the past few days declared that fall was upon us. Crisp, cold nights and cool, pleasant days. The change in seasons usually brought a change in the types of complaints and problems we saw in the ER, and this year was no exception. The sunburns, cuts, and tick bites of summer were giving way to colds and coughs and a few cases of pneumonia.

Lori walked out of triage, leading a young man who apparently had not checked his calendar. He wore flip-flops, dirt-smudged bathing trunks, and a much-used Clemson T-shirt. Streaks of blood coursed down his forehead, drawing my eyes to the treble fishhook embedded firmly in his scalp. His sheepish grin was a combination of embarrassment and a significant number of adult libations.

"Minor trauma." Lori shook her head and continued down the hallway.

As I tossed the chart of the asthmatic in room 3 into the discharge basket, the EMS phone squawked to life.

"ER, this is EMS 1!"

It was Denton Roberts, and the voice of the usually calm and collected paramedic was high-pitched and strained. Amy Connors glanced up at me. She rolled her chair over to the phone and flipped the receiver onto speaker mode.

"This is the ER, EMS 1. Go ahead."

The phone crackled loudly and Amy flinched, moving her head away.

"Is the doctor nearby?"

Amy looked up at me again. "Dr. Lesslie is standing right here. Go ahead."

"Dr. Lesslie, this is Denton Roberts. We're about ten minutes out with a three-year-old boy drowning...or *near* drowning."

Amy's eyes widened. Lori Davidson had walked up behind me. She slid the chart of our fishhook patient onto the countertop, then turned and headed into cardiac.

"What have you got, Denton?" I was leaning over the counter and staring down at the receiver.

"A three-year-old, like I said, Doc. His babysitter found him in the deep end of the swimming pool. The kid was at the bottom, and it took her a while to get him out. Don't know how long he was in the water. When we got there, he didn't have a pulse, but she was doing chest compressions and we took over."

There was mumbling in the background and Denton was hollering to someone, maybe his partner.

"Sorry, Doc, it's crazy here. A bunch of neighbors came over, and the parents just arrived. Anyway, we're loaded and pulling out of the driveway now. He's intubated but we're not going to be able to get a line started."

"Is he breathing? Any pulse?"

"Nothin'."

The word hung in the air, and I glanced over at Amy. Her youngest boy was three, maybe four. She looked away.

"Cardiac when you get here. We'll get things ready."

"Roger that. Cardiac on arrival. And Doc, he's been down a long time." The receiver fell silent and I headed across the hall.

"Respiratory therapy is on the way down," Amy called after me. "Lab and X-ray too."

"Thanks."

Lori had her back to the door and stood beside the stretcher, readying equipment and supplies on the counter.

"Doesn't sound very promising," I told her.

She turned and stood up straight. There was a deep sigh and then, "Three years old, right?"

"That's what Denton said."

She stood there for a moment, looking down at the syringes in her hand. "He's going to make it."

We always tried to be optimistic, to hope for the best, but there was something in her voice that made me look at her.

"What do you—"

The pneumatic hissing of the ambulance-entrance doors announced the arrival of EMS 1 and I didn't finish my question. Within a minute they were rolling into the room and the quiet calm exploded into chaotic but organized activity.

"Still no pulse." Denton's face was beet-red and dripping with sweat. He was hunched over the limp, lifeless body of the little boy. The paramedic continued his chest compressions, not missing a beat as we moved the child to our bed.

Denton had intubated him as soon as he arrived at the scene and I checked to confirm the clear, plastic airway was in the right place. Water continued to gurgle up into the tube and was suctioned away as soon as it appeared.

"He was full, Doc. We've tried to clear him out the best we could."

"Has he ever had any sign of life?" I looked over at the paramedic and then down at the boy.

"No, nothing. His color's been okay, but no effort at breathing or any cardiac activity."

The door opened and an X-ray tech wheeled a portable machine into the room.

"Chest X-ray?" She maneuvered the awkward equipment to the edge of the stretcher. Before I could answer, a young man and woman burst into the room.

"BJ! Is he alive?"

Lori looked over at me, her eyes wide. I nodded and turned to the couple.

The man froze halfway to the bed. His previously flushed face now drained of all color as he looked down at the little boy. His wild eyes scanned the room and his hands began to tremble.

I got the attention of Denton's partner and motioned with my head to a chair in the corner. He immediately went over to the father, took him by the shoulders, and guided him away from the bed.

"Let's have a seat over here, sir. You need to get off your feet and take some deep breaths."

The young woman had rushed to the stretcher and flung herself across the body of her son.

"BJ!" she wailed. "BJ!"

Lori put a hand gently on the woman's shoulder. "Ma'am, step over here with me. We need to be able to work on your son."

The mother slowly stood, one of her hands slowly trailing across the boy's shoulder and down his right arm.

Denton had somehow managed to continue his chest compressions. He looked up at me, wet hair matted to his forehead, and then glanced at the cardiac monitor.

"What's that?"

I followed his gaze to the small, green screen. Nothing. Just an undulating lifeless line.

"I don't see—"

There it was. One small blip on the monitor, and then another.

"Has he had any of that before?"

"No," Denton shook his head. "He's been flatline the whole time."

There were a few more erratic blips, spaced between painfully long pauses. Then they became more frequent, almost organized.

"Any pulse with that?" I continued bagging the child, making sure his chest was rising with each squeeze.

Denton stopped compressing BJ's chest. He placed one hand over the boy's heart and two fingers over his left carotid artery.

A hushed silence fell over the room as we all looked first at Denton, then at the monitor, and then back to Denton.

His eyes were closed, squeezed shut as stood over the boy. Slowly he began to nod his head.

"I've got something."

The boy's mother let out a loud gasp.

The paramedic opened his eyes and looked over at the monitor. The blips had become regular now, with a rate of about a 100 beats a minute.

"I can feel a pulse with each of those complexes," he told me.

I had been watching Denton and the monitor, and for a second I stopped bagging the boy. I was about to deliver another inspiration, when BJ's chest jerked and air rushed through the tube.

I removed the ambu bag from the tube and watched as the boy took a breath, and then another.

"He's breathing!" His father jumped up from the chair and bounded over to the side of the stretcher. "I saw it, he's breathing!"

An hour later, BJ and his parents were on the way up to the ICU. He still had a pulse and a good blood pressure. And he was still breathing on his own.

'How do you explain that, Doc?" Denton was helping us straighten up the room and was restocking his emergency supplies. "He was under water for at least five minutes, maybe more."

"You said the water was cold," I ventured, wondering the same question.

"It was freezing. Apparently they get the water from a well, and the nights have been cold. That's supposed to help, I know, but...do you think he's going to be okay? I mean his brain and everything."

"He was making purposeful movements and was starting to look around," I answered. "Those are good signs. And when you consider the condition he was in when you found him, and when he got here...It usually doesn't turn out this way."

"He's going to be okay."

There was that tone of voice again, that assurance. Denton and I spun around and looked at Lori. Her back was to us as she organized supplies on the countertop.

She slowly turned and faced us.

"Something told me, and I just know. He's going to be fine."

THE *Miracle* OF ANSWERED PRAYER

The LORD is near to all who call on him,
to all who call on him in truth,
He fulfills the desires of those who fear him;
He hears their cry and saves them.

PSALM 145:18-19

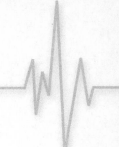

Chauncey Taylor

Ida Fleming was in room 3, gasping for breath and barely clinging to life. Again.

She was eighty-three years old and her failing heart brought her into the ER once or twice a month. This was the third time in four weeks. Things were getting worse.

"Ida, if we can't turn things around pretty quickly, I'm afraid you're going to have to go back on a ventilator."

She looked at me with kind, fearless eyes, and nodded her head.

Lori Davidson had started an IV and was pushing some medicine. Hopefully this would improve things, but we would soon reach the point where nothing we did was going to help.

Always cheerful, always calm, Ida had been in and out of the ER and the hospital since I'd begun working in Rock Hill. It was impossible not to be drawn to such a beautiful spirit. She was a rare woman.

Several years earlier, I had seen her in the ER when she was *not* short of breath. She wasn't a patient, but had ridden in the back of an ambulance with her twenty-five-year-old grandson, Chauncey Taylor. He had been involved in a drug deal gone bad, been shot twice in the belly, and had dragged himself onto her front porch. Bleeding and stoned on an assortment of illegal substances, he had pounded on the wooden deck until she came to the door.

Chauncey nearly died that day. Most of his blood was left behind on Ida's porch, and we barely got him to the OR in time. Ida had been standing beside him in major trauma when I walked back into the room. The nurse stepped out into the hallway, and it was just the three of us.

"Doctor, if you don't mind, I'm going to pray."

I stepped over beside her, rested both hands on the stretcher rail, and closed my eyes. What followed was a woman of faith talking with her Lord. No pretense, no flowery language or lofty petitions. She asked the Lord to save the life of her grandson. And believing and knowing he was going to do that, she asked him to change his life. She asked him to lead Chauncey away from drugs and alcohol, and from the company of his so-called friends who "brought him to low places." Then she patted the unresponsive Chauncey on his shoulder and uttered a simple yet promise-claiming "Amen."

Chauncey survived his gunshots and lived. It took him a while to get back on his feet, but when he did, it was the same old thing—drugs, alcohol, and the law.

We treated him for a variety of problems over the next couple of years. Drug overdoses, chest pain from snorting cocaine, two or three DUIs involving injuries to other drivers. And there were stab wounds on at least two occasions, though no more gunshots. Everyone in the ER knew him, as did everyone on the police force. He was bad news.

Sometimes, when I hadn't seen him for a couple of months, and when Ida was in the ER and could talk, I would ask her about her grandson. She never failed to smile at the mention of his name, and to begin nodding her head.

"Not so good just yet, Dr. Lesslie. But the Lord is going to change that young man. I pray for that every morning and every night. It's going to happen—just hasn't happened yet."

Then one day there was a chance, a real opportunity for Chauncey to turn things around. He was involved in a minor burglary and was sentenced to eight months in jail. He would be away from his friends and his drugs and would be offered counseling for his substance abuse. Ida was hopeful this would be the turning point.

When he was released, he told her he had seen the light and was going to mend his ways. No more drugs, no more alcohol. He was even going to stop smoking and get a job.

That lasted four days. He was soon right back where he had been.

"It's just so hard to turn away from that kind of life," Ida had told me. "Just so hard. But I'm prayin'."

He was paying a steep price for his chosen lifestyle, not only with the heartache he caused his family and Ida, but also in his own body. One morning I picked up the clipboard for room 2 and saw his name, and then his complaint—"sick." I pulled the curtain aside and was shocked by what I saw. He had lost twenty or thirty pounds and was jaundiced—a deep orange color. His IV drug use had given him hepatitis B and the virus had nearly destroyed his liver. Chauncey *was* "sick" this time, and he nearly died. Just before he was released from the hospital, I visited him upstairs on one of the medical floors.

"This is it, Doc. I'm done with drugs, and with alcohol. I don't want to go out like this. Done. I swear I am."

His grandmother was sitting in the corner of the room, looking over at her Chauncey and smiling. Hope springs eternal, but I was afraid I knew better.

We didn't see Chauncey Taylor in the ER for a long time and didn't hear a word about him. Months passed, and Ida came in a couple of times, her heart continuing to weaken, each visit worse than the last.

Finally it happened. EMS called in a cardiac arrest—it was Ida. She had managed to get to her phone and dial 9-1-1 and had then collapsed onto the living room floor as she hung up the receiver. We tried everything, and worked with her for almost an hour, but she was gone.

The paramedics and respiratory therapist left the cardiac room, and Lori and I were alone with her. We stood in silence beside the stretcher, gazing down at this remarkable woman. She was finally at peace—no more shortness of breath, no more near brushes with death.

The door opened and closed behind us, but we didn't look up. Slow, deliberate footsteps made their way to the stretcher. Sure and steady hands grabbed the rail opposite us, and we looked up into the face of Chauncey Taylor.

He smiled at us, then reached out and gently caressed the top of his grandmother's head.

I studied the man, first noticing the clothes he was wearing. Neat, clean—something unusual for Chauncey. And then I looked at his face. He had gained some weight, and his color was good. He looked healthy.

"I didn't make it in time," he whispered, his voice low, reverent.

"It all happened so fast," Lori told him. "She wouldn't have known you were here."

He gazed at his grandmother and then his eyes found mine. "She knows." He was still whispering, and slowly nodded his head. "She knows."

"She was a great woman," I told him. "We'll miss her."

"She saved my life, Doc. It's because of her that I've been clean for six months. And it's because of her that I'm going to stay clean."

I searched his eyes and wanted to believe him. No, I *did* believe him.

Your Will—Not Mine

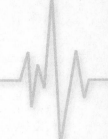

Tuesday, 6:35 a.m. Lori slumped into a chair and folded her arms across her chest. She sat there for a moment then sighed and shook her head. "I need some help."

I glanced around the department and checked the patient ID board. The department was empty. Our shift was just beginning, and Virginia Granger and I had been sitting at the nurses' station when Lori had walked over. We both looked at her and waited. It was rare for our "resident helper" to ask for help.

Amy Connors, our unit secretary, walked up and deftly moved her chair back with one knee. She carefully set a cardboard container holding four steaming cups of coffee on the desktop and sat down. She had heard Lori's words, and now turned to the nurse and said, "What's up?"

Lori sighed again. "It's one of my closest friends, Kelly. We went to grade school and high school together. We were bridesmaids in each other's weddings. A little over six months ago, Kelly found out her sister has ovarian cancer. Thirty-two years old, and the doctors told her nothing could be done. It was too far advanced."

"Wow, that's quick," Amy said quietly. "I'm sorry."

"It's been hard on everybody," Lori continued. "But especially Kelly. She was the older sister, the role model. Whenever her sister got hurt or got into trouble, Kelly was there to fix it." She paused and looked down at the floor. "She can't fix it this time."

We sat in silence for a moment, and I thought about this disease we call *cancer*—the "crab." It comes in many forms, but not many more aggressive, merciless, or ruthless than ovarian cancer. The diagnosis is usually made at a point when the illness is long past being treatable.

Virginia Granger rolled her chair closer to Lori and leaned forward. "What can we do?"

43

Lori took a deep breath and looked at her head nurse.

"Kelly has been crushed by this, and she called me last night in tears. She was angry."

"Anger is part of the process," I interjected. "And it might be good if—"

"There's nothing good about it." Lori glanced at me, her eyes wet with tears. "She's mad at God for allowing this to happen. But more than that, she's mad that he doesn't answer their prayers about this. The whole family and their church have been in constant prayer since the diagnosis, and her sister just gets weaker every day, and the pain is getting worse, and she…"

Lori's voice broke and her head slumped to her chest.

"And she called to ask you 'Why?'" Virginia said gently. "You've been *her* big sister all these years, and she wants you to fix things, or at least explain them."

Lori sobbed and nodded.

Silence again, except for Lori's pained breaths. Amy handed her a box of Kleenex from the countertop.

A minute or two passed and she looked up at us.

"How do you answer that question? How do you begin to explain why God is not healing her sister? I don't know what to tell her."

Virginia leaned back in her chair, crossed her legs, and began drumming the armrests with her long, slender fingers.

Amy looked over at her and tilted her head to one side.

The head nurse took a deep breath and the drumming stopped. "Lori, as sure as I'm sitting right here, I know the Lord doesn't rejoice in our suffering. But in the ER there's pain and heartache all around us—every day." She paused but her eyes never left Lori's. "The Lord is not blind to *any* of this."

Lori leaned forward in her chair. "But Kelly's family—all of them—are Christians, followers of Jesus. And if *their* prayers aren't answered, then…" Her voice was pleading, and it broke off again in soft sobs.

"How do you know they aren't being answered?" Virginia was peering over the top of her bifocals, her eyes soft, motherlike. I had never seen here like this before.

"Let me tell you what I've learned about prayer," she continued.

Virginia had an older brother, Michael, and the two had been very close during their school years and into their twenties. They lived a few hours apart but managed to see each other on a frequent basis. He found a niche in the insurance business and she pursued her career in nursing.

"I always took it for granted that we would be close, that our relationship would always be solid, special. And it *was*, up until ten or eleven years ago. Something happened—I can't even remember what exactly—and we had an argument. I suppose it was the wrong time and the wrong place, but things escalated and words were spoken—hurtful words—things that should never have been said. But they were, and our relationship exploded. Looking back on it now, I don't…"

She paused, folded her hands, and shook her head.

"Anyway." Virginia sat up straight in her chair and adjusted her eyeglasses. "That was that, for a lot of years. We didn't talk, we didn't write, we didn't see each other. And I grieved for the loss of my brother. This went on for years. We might bump into each other at a family gathering, but there was no real communication, no sign on his part of being sorry." She chuckled and shook her head again. "Nor on mine, I suppose. But I was praying every day. I asked the Lord to heal our relationship, to soften Michael's heart. But nothing happened. No phone call, no letter. Nothing. But I kept praying for the Lord to intervene. I *knew* this could change, that it *had* to change, if only Michael could see the truth. Then he got sick."

Suddenly, I remembered. Virginia didn't talk about her personal life very much, but a few years ago she'd told me that her brother had been ill. She hadn't mentioned his name or what kind of problem he was having. It was another one of our longtime nurses, Harriet Gray, who had told me he had died. Harriet was a year younger than Virginia and was her closest friend. Virginia missed a day of work to go to his funeral, and that was it.

"It was terminal," Virginia said bluntly. "When I heard, he was already at home, dying. There was nothing else to be done for him. I threw some stuff in a bag, jumped in my car, and headed out to see him. I remember saying a prayer, asking that he not have to suffer, and I prayed once again that his heart would be open and we would be able to talk, before he…"

She looked over at Lori and their eyes met. Virginia smiled and said, "I knew right then, right in that instant, that the Lord had answered my prayer. But it wasn't at all what I had been hoping and praying for. He had softened *my* heart. *That* was the work that needed to be done and he had done it. All those years, praying for Michael to see the light, and it was *my* eyes that had been closed—*my* eyes that had been blind—*my* heart that had been hardened. The Lord was answering my prayers, and he was waiting for me to understand." She stopped and put a hand on Lori's shoulder.

"But Ms. Granger, I don't know…" Lori's voice trailed off and her head slumped to her chest again.

"That's the point, Lori." Virginia's voice was strong and sure. "Most of the time we *don't* know. We just have to believe and trust. We may not understand the things that are happening around us—happening *to* us—but we have to believe that his ultimate will is for our good, to bring us closer to him. And we have to keep praying. He'll answer those prayers—every one of them. The important thing is to trust those answers, to learn to accept *his* will. He sees what we can't. He knows what we don't. It's hard sometimes, but our walk on *this* earth is full of things we don't want, and things we don't expect."

The ambulance-entrance doors flew open and a young woman ran into the department. In her arms was a young child, two or three years old, his face a dusky blue. He wasn't breathing.

"Somebody help me!" she screamed, her eyes wide with fear. "Lord, save my baby!"

We all jumped up at the same instant. But it was Lori who turned the corner of the nurses' station first.

"Let's go!"

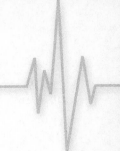

Without Ceasing

"Now *that's* an answer to prayer." Lori Davidson was smiling, watching the ambulance-entrance doors close behind Darren Whipple.

She took a deep breath and turned back to the chart on the counter.

"Darren? An answer to prayer?" Darren Whipple had been one of my partners for more than a dozen years, and I had just relieved him from his overnight shift. *What prayer was he an answer to?*

Lori put her pen down and looked over at me.

"Can't you tell the difference? Don't you think he's—"

"Easier to get along with." Virginia Granger interrupted the nurse and walked over beside us. "Yes, he's easier to get along with," she repeated.

"That's not what I…" Lori faltered. "Yes, he's easier to get along with, but I meant he seems to be…nicer—different."

"Wait a minute." I turned and faced the two women. "What's going on here? What are we talking about?"

"We're talking about your partner, Darren Whipple." Virginia peered at me over her bifocals. "Don't tell me you've been unaware of the problems we've had of late."

"Problems? With Darren again? I thought that was resolved months ago, when I had that long talk with him."

Virginia frowned and shook her head. "Apparently your little talk didn't have the effect you thought it did. Or maybe it just didn't stick."

Darren Whipple was a well-trained and efficient emergency physician. He had joined us right out of his residency and immediately fit in with the ER and medical staff. His "claim to fame," as he referred to it, was that his great-grandfather had been a famous surgeon and had had an intricate abdominal surgical procedure named after him.

"I have an uncle nicknamed 'Bones,'" Amy Connors had said when she first heard this story. "Does that make *me* famous?"

Darren quickly came to understand the secretary's unusual sense of humor, and the two became good friends. In fact, Darren seemed to be friends with everyone in the department.

That began to change about a year ago. There was not one particular instance, or individual patient that seemed to trigger things, but Darren gradually became more distant, quieter. "Distracted" was the word Virginia had used.

Over a few months, all the signs began to declare themselves: physical and emotional exhaustion, cynicism, detachment, doubt about what he was doing and why. Virginia was the first to see and understand. It took me longer. Darren was burning out.

—————

"Dr. Whipple, here are the labs you requested." The young lab tech put the slips of paper on the counter next to the chart of the cardiac patient. Darren was standing there, running streams of heart tracings through his fingers, searching for some clue as to why this man was having blackouts.

The tech had almost made it to the door when Whipple yelled at her.

"Where are his electrolytes? I need to know his sodium and potassium!"

She turned, ducked her head, and mumbled, "Dr. Whipple, you didn't order electrolytes. You only ordered—"

"I most certainly ordered them! What's the matter with you? I'm trying to take care of this man and you're…you're…Oh, get out of here!"

The tech backpedaled, broke into tears, and scurried down the hall.

Darren looked at his wide-eyed patient, grabbed the clipboard, and stomped out of the room and over to the nurses' station.

"Here." He handed the clipboard of cardiac to the doctor working with him. "I need to take a break." He stalked down the hallway and disappeared into our lounge.

That was the first of several quickly recurring episodes. Invariably Darren would lose his temper, blow up over some trivial issue, and yell at a tech or staff member, frequently bringing them to tears.

It was a radical change in his behavior, and we all noticed it.

"When are you going to talk with Dr. Whipple? He's really messin' up."
Amy was not known to mince her words and was obviously concerned
about her friend. "Not just here, but at home too. He told me the other
night that things were rough with his wife. 'Difficult,' I think he said."

A few days later, I came in early to relieve him.

"Let's go back to the lounge for a few minutes," I told him. "We need
to talk."

We spent the next forty-five minutes discussing his recent "difficul-
ties." At first he was defensive, but gradually he began to listen. We were
concerned about him, and wanted him to be happy—at peace. At present,
that wasn't the case, and it was affecting the entire department.

"Burnout is a common problem among those of us in medicine," I told
him. "Especially ER docs. Long hours, difficult and complex patients, hol-
idays, nights, weekends. And only an infrequent thank-you. You've been
doing this more than ten years, and that seems to be the breaking point.
Somebody either figures out how to carry on in a meaningful, productive
way, or they do something different. I think that's where you are, Darren."

He had lowered his head and was silent for a moment.

"Robert," he finally said. "This is what I love to do. I've just got to get
things together. Thanks for talking with me."

We discussed counseling, fewer hours, more exercise, more time with
his family. He was going to try all those things.

Every week or so I would ask how he was doing—was he making prog-
ress? The answer was always the same: "I'm doing fine." Finally I stopped
asking. I was hopeful this was going to work—hopeful that this would be
a turning point for Darren Whipple.

Apparently it wasn't.

—————

"Let's talk about this 'answer to prayer' business, Lori. What exactly
do you mean?"

Virginia glanced at me, adjusted her glasses, and headed for her office.

"It's just that I've been praying a long time for Dr. Whipple," Lori began.
"He's such a nice man and a good doctor—I hate to see him so tormented.

I think the talk you had with him helped some, but like Virginia said, it didn't stick. He was better, or seemed to be. But something was simmering just below the surface. There was something in his eyes, some unrest or something. I just sensed he could explode at any minute. He was trying hard, but it was too much for him. And then he *did* explode."

"Explode? What are you talking about?" This was news to me.

"Ms. Granger made me promise not to say anything to you." Lori glanced around the department and lowered her voice. "She made Dr. Whipple promise too, and Sharon Mahaffey."

"Sharon Mahaffey? What does she have to do with any of this?" Sharon was a veteran ER nurse and worked the night shift.

"Dr. Whipple blew up at Sharon one night and she went straight to Ms. Granger. She said she didn't have to take the abuse that Dr. Whipple gave her and would resign from the ER if something didn't happen."

"Why didn't I hear anything about this?" I shook my head, wondering what planet I had been on.

"Like I said, Ms. Granger made us all swear to keep it quiet. She wanted to see if Dr. Whipple could change and make things right."

She paused and looked at me. "I'm sorry, Dr. Lesslie, if—"

"No, I understand, Lori. If Virginia wanted to keep this quiet, you were only doing what she asked. But what happened?"

She shook her head and again glanced around the department.

"The four of us were in her office and she had Dr. Whipple sit down, right in front of her. She told him that his behavior was unacceptable, that he needed to decide if he wanted to work in this ER or whether he wanted to be a doctor at all. That really got his attention, but he didn't say anything. He just sat there and listened. Then Ms. Granger stopped, and we all sat there for a couple of minutes, no one saying a word. Finally, she got up, walked over to Dr. Whipple, and put a hand on his shoulder. She told him we're a family, and a family looks after each other. We wanted to look after him, but he had to decide something first. He had to decide if he wanted to be in this family.

"I think I saw tears in his eyes, but he looked down and I couldn't be sure. When he sat up, it was like a light had been turned on. He apologized to Ms. Granger and Sharon, and he apologized to me. He thanked us, then walked out of the office and back to work. He's been different ever since, as I said a little while ago. But he's not just easier to get along with—he's happier and more at peace. I bet when he gets the chance, he'll apologize to you too. You'll see. He's different."

She stopped and smiled at me.

"I see what you mean by an 'answer to prayer,'" I said quietly. "You've been praying a long time for this, and your prayers have been answered."

"Answered in the form of Virginia Granger," Lori chuckled. "Funny how the Lord works sometimes. He knew just what Dr. Whipple needed to hear and when he needed to hear it. And he knew who he needed to hear it from. He used Ms. Granger to answer my prayers."

I glanced at Virginia's closed office door, and again at Lori—thankful for these two wise women the Lord had placed in my life.

Unseen *Miracles*

*A farmer went out to sow his seed.
As he was scattering the seed, some fell along the path,
and the birds came and ate it up. Some fell on rocky places,
where it did not have much soil. It sprang up quickly,
because the soil was shallow. But when the sun came up,
the plants were scorched, and they withered because they
had no root. Other seed fell among thorns, which grew
up and choked the plants. Still other seed fell on good
soil, where it produced a crop—a hundred, sixty or thirty
times what was sown. Whoever has ears, let them hear.*

Jesus, in Matthew 13:3-9

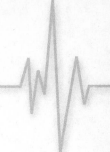

A Seed Planted

Harriet Gray's glass was always half full, and if she had a motto to live by, it would probably have been "accentuate the positive, eliminate the negative...don't mess with Mr. In-Between." She lived that way, and spent forty-two years as a nurse in the ER demonstrating those words with her infectious smile, her warm caring, and a crushing hug that left little doubt how she felt about you. If you could paint the picture of a grandmother, it would be Harriet Gray.

She and Virginia Granger had been together in the trenches of the ER for several decades and were each other's best friend. When Virginia's husband had died a few years ago, Harriet was right beside her, day and night, for more than a week. And when Harriet lost consciousness in the ER one day with new-onset diabetes, it was Virginia's turn. She stayed in the ICU with Harriet until she was finally able to move to a regular bed.

Together they trained a lot of nurses and molded a lot of young physicians who worked in the ER. I was fortunate enough to be one of those young ER docs, and fortunate enough to have the air hugged out of me on numerous occasions.

Jackie Watts was lying on the stretcher of the cardiac room, eyes closed, arms folded over his abdomen. He had been brought in from the county jail, complaining of chest pain. Two sheriff's deputies had accompanied him.

"Ain't nothin' wrong with him, Doc," one of the deputies told me. A wad of snuff under his upper lip made it hard to understand him, and I leaned closer and watched his mouth, intrigued. "Says he has chest pain, but he was doin' fine. Heck, he's twenty-six years old. He ain't havin' no heart attack."

We were standing in the hallway just outside cardiac, waiting for one of our techs to finish an EKG.

"He's probably just lookin' for a chance to—"

There was a metallic crash, followed by a high-pitched scream. The young tech flew out of the room, her eyes wide and mouth gaping. She jabbed a finger behind her, pointing into cardiac, and ran down the hallway, disappearing around the far corner.

"What tha—" The deputy jumped back and his hand flew to the handle of his holstered gun.

Then it was Jackie's turn. He bolted through the doorway—EKG electrodes and wires dangling from his chest and arms—and right into the enormous belly of the deputy. The law officer didn't budge, but Jackie, weighing two hundred pounds less, bounced off and collapsed on the floor. He shook his head, glanced around the room, and was about to get up when the officer stepped over and put two heavy hands on his shoulders.

"Hold on right there, Jackie. You ain't goin' nowhere."

The other deputy hurried over to the scene of the near escape, and the two of them lifted Jackie off the floor and carried him over to the stretcher. This time he was handcuffed to the rails—both arms and both legs. He wasn't going anywhere.

"Oh! My chest!" he wailed.

"Yeah, right." One of the deputies smirked. "You'd better behave, Jackie. Next time you try that, we won't be so nice."

Jackie cocked an eye at him, opened his mouth to say something, but remained silent. He closed his eyes again and folded his arms over his belly.

"Do what you gotta do, Doc," the portly deputy told me in the hallway. "I know you need to check out his chest pain, but we'd like to get back to the jail as soon as we can. We'll be right outside if you need us."

"It shouldn't take long. We'll let you know."

We *would* have to check out his complaints—at least finish the EKG we'd started. Probably going to have to find another tech to do that.

His vital signs were completely normal. His physical exam, other than a multitude of tattoos, was unremarkable. And his EKG was fine. We would soon be releasing him into the loving care of the deputies.

I was at the nurses' station, finishing up his chart, when Harriet Gray walked out of cardiac and over to where I stood.

"Troubled young man, Mr. Jackie." She was smiling, but her furrowed brow betrayed her real emotion. "Troubled."

She walked over to the medicine room and disappeared through the doorway.

I walked into cardiac to give Mr. Watts the good news. We were alone, and before I could say anything, he blurted, "Who was that woman? That old nurse who was just in here?"

His eyes were narrow slits and his fists were clenched, struggling against the handcuffs. My face flushed and anger spread through me like a searing wave. He was talking about Harriet.

"That's *nurse* Gray. She—"

"I don't want her in here again! Do you hear me? Keep her away from me!"

It was all I could do to remain calm and not get right down in his face.

"You hear me?" he screamed again.

I walked out of the room and through the ambulance entrance. The two deputies were leaning against the front hood of their patrol car and stood up straight as I walked over.

"Your prisoner is ready to go, guys. You were right. There's nothing wrong with him. Nothing we can fix."

Jackie Watts continued to follow the path of too many young men in this town—in a lot of towns. We would see him every couple of months, usually in the company of city or county officers, and with an assortment of injuries and ailments. He had a few stab wounds, broken bones, and at least two overdoses. And then he just disappeared. Several years went by, and he didn't darken our doorstep.

Then one day he appeared again. This time he came walking through the triage room with Lori Davidson, right up to where I stood. I recognized him immediately, and took a step backward.

"Doc, you remember me? I'm Jackie Watts."

"He said it was important, Dr. Lesslie," Lori said from behind the man, raising her eyebrows and shrugging. "That it would only take a minute. I hope it's okay."

"Sure, Lori." I nodded at her, then looked at Jackie. He was standing straight, freshly shaven and neatly dressed. Not the way I last saw him. "What can I do for you, Mr. Watts?"

"Is nurse Gray here?" he asked, his voice quiet and his eyes searching the department. "I think that's her name."

Lori's face flushed. She quickly turned around and walked back out to triage.

"Harriet Gray?" I remembered his outburst and wondered what in the world was on his mind. And whether it was good.

"Yes, I think so. The…large nurse, gray-headed?"

"That would be Harriet," I nodded, studying his eyes. They continued to wander around the area and finally locked on mine.

"I…I need to talk with her. For just a moment."

We stood there, looking at each other. *What does this man want?*

"I'm afraid that won't be possible, Mr. Watts."

"She doesn't work here anymore?" His shoulders slumped and he started looking around again.

"No, she died a couple of weeks ago."

He froze, let out a long, loud sigh, and stared at the floor.

"I should have come sooner. I…"

"Is there anything I can help you with?"

Jackie Watts looked up at me, his eyes softened now, and a smile began to form on his face.

"I've been in prison, Doc. For the last three years. Best thing that could have ever happened to me. Not at first, though. I was a real troublemaker, I guess you'd say. But I started thinkin', and wonderin' what the rest of my life was gonna be like. And then I started thinkin' about what nurse Gray told me, that day I was over in that room, handcuffed to the bed."

He turned and pointed to cardiac.

"You remember that day, Doc?"

"I remember, Jackie."

"She got me pretty upset, and you were gettin' upset with me, the way I was carrying on. The reason was, I didn't like what she was tellin' me. She wasn't yellin' at me or anything. I just didn't like what she was sayin'. But you know what? I never forgot it. Never. I started thinkin' about it in prison, and every day, I repeated her words. She told me, 'Jackie, you're better than this. But don't worry, the Lord's not finished with you yet.' And you know what, Doc? He wasn't. And he's still not. I'm doin' fine now, and just wanted to come by and…" He paused and took a deep breath, tears glistening in his eyes. "And let her know. At least I got to tell you. And I'm thankful for that."

We stood there, silent, and I knew what he needed. But it was Amy who got out of her chair, walked around the desk, and grabbed Jackie. She locked him in a tight, suffocating hug.

"This is from Harriet."

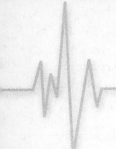

Burning Bridges

"What happened this time?" I recognized the name on the chart Lori Davidson dropped into the "to be seen" basket.

Toby Bridges—busted lip.

"Another fight." She sighed and shook her head. "Of course it wasn't his fault, just like it never is. Said he had to step in and defend one of his friends. The problem was the other guy had a pool stick in his hand and hit Toby in the mouth with it. I don't see any teeth missing, but it's going to take awhile to put back together."

Toby was well known to the ER staff. The seventeen-year-old had carved out a troubling path during his teenage years, frequently ending up in the emergency department with an assortment of injuries, and frequently with an entourage of uniformed officers. He was bright and should have figured things out by now. His parents, both professionals, had tried everything—counseling, military school, tough love, really tough love. Nothing was working. Toby Bridges was headed for trouble.

"Alright, I'll go get started."

Lori handed the clipboard to me. "He's been drinking again."

I glanced at the clock over the ambulance entrance—*4:32 p.m.*—and shook my head.

Toby was lying on the far-right stretcher in minor trauma and holding a piece of cotton gauze to his injured mouth.

"Hello, Dr. Lesslie." His speech was slurred, and I wasn't sure if it was the gauze or the alcohol or both.

"Hello, Toby. Lori tells me you've been in another tussle."

The nurse had a suture tray ready beside his stretcher, and I sat down on a stool and rolled over next to him.

"I didn't see that pool stick." He mumbled, shook his head, and took the gauze away from his mangled lip. Lori was right—it was going to take awhile to put this back together.

⁓

Toby was fourteen years old when I first saw him in the ER. His mother and two police officers brought him in. He and a couple of friends had decided to break into a neighbor's house but hadn't planned on the alarm system and the quick response of a nearby squad car. The approaching siren had caused the boys to panic, and Toby ran through the sliding glass door leading onto the back porch. It shattered, leaving him with several large, deep gashes of his wrists and forearms. *That* took awhile to put back together too.

A close family friend in town happened to be an attorney and was able to shield Toby from any serious charges.

"I'm not sure we're doing the boy any favor here," she told his parents. "He needs to get his act straight, but he also doesn't need something like this on his record."

The next time Toby wasn't as fortunate. He was fifteen years old when EMS brought him to the ER late one night.

"The kid's beat up pretty bad," Denton told me. He and his partner were moving Toby onto the stretcher in major trauma. "Whoever did this rolled him in a ditch and left him for dead. A truck driver just happened to catch a glimpse of what he thought was a body and called it in. He's mighty lucky."

"Don't know if I'd call him lucky."

Denton and I twisted around. Detective Terry Jamison was standing in the doorway with his arms folded across his chest. He was casually chewing on the end of a yellow pencil.

"100 over 60," Lori told us. "Pupils equal but sluggish. Doesn't respond much to pain."

My attention refocused on the injured teenager. We spent the next hour getting him stabilized and determining the extent of his injuries—three fractured ribs, a fractured jaw, a bruised spleen, and a closed-head injury. He was starting to wake up and was trying to speak.

"I'd like to ask him a few questions when he's able." Detective Jamison stood at the foot of the stretcher, drumming a notepad with his pencil.

"Probably going to be a little while, Terry," I told him. "What do you know about this?"

"We've got a pretty good idea about who beat him, but we need his confirmation. Looks like a drug deal gone bad. My guess is that he was trying to score some marijuana and stiffed the wrong people. If it's who we think it is, these guys are bad actors. But they're not stupid. They left a bag of weed in his pants pocket, enough for him to be charged as a dealer. Like I said, I don't know if I'd call this kid lucky."

He wasn't. He recovered from his injuries, but was unable to avoid the long arm of the law. He spent some time in juvenile detention, but was soon out and quickly back to his old ways. If ever a young man was destined for a bad ending, it was Toby Bridges.

Two months after I sewed up his lip, EMS brought him to the ER again. This time it looked as if he had reached that bad ending.

Toby had lost his driver's license and was driving a friend's pickup when he lost control, crossed the median, and hit an SUV. He was on a backboard when the paramedics wheeled him into the department.

"What's he got?" Lori asked Denton Roberts.

"We put him in spinal protocol as a precaution," the paramedic answered. "Looks like he has a forehead laceration but that's it—nothing else that we could find. The driver of the other vehicle was not so lucky. Broken femur and maybe a couple of ribs. He was helicoptered to Charlotte."

"Wass goin' on?"

Toby reeked of alcohol and his glazed eyes wandered around the room. Denton looked at Lori and shook his head. "Where do you want him?"

"I guess take him to minor, bed C. The only problem is Ezekiel Stevenson is back there with his grandchild. But there's no other bed available."

The African Methodist Episcopal churches had a big presence in Rock Hill, and Ezekiel was the minister of one of them. He had just brought one of his grandchildren in with a shoulder injury. The eight-year-old girl probably had a broken collarbone, the result of one of an orthopedist's best friends—a trampoline.

"Let's just hope he behaves himself," Lori added.

"Wass goin' on?"

By the time we finished taking care of Toby, Ezekiel and his grand-daughter were gone. Toby was able to stand, talk, and walk out of the department with two police officers, his hands cuffed behind his back. He was facing serious jail time.

―――

Five years passed before I saw Toby Bridges again, once more in major trauma. It was a gunshot to the chest, and I called for a stat portable X-ray.

"Already on the way." Lori had started one IV and was working on another.

The door to major opened and the portable machine lumbered into the room, guided by one of the radiology techs.

"Start with a chest," I said, glancing at the tech. "And—"

Lori looked up at me and then followed my stare. Her jaw dropped.

It was Toby Bridges, dressed in the neat white jacket and slacks of a radiology technician.

He smiled at us and maneuvered the machine to the side of the stretcher. With quiet expertise, he positioned the cassette under the patient's chest, shot the film, and hurried out of the room.

Later, we had a chance to talk.

"When did this happen, Toby?" I pointed to his hospital name tag.

"I started at the General a couple of days ago, Dr. Lesslie. Finished my training at York Tech and wanted to work here."

I nodded and studied his eyes. This was a different Toby Bridges—a changed Toby Bridges.

He smiled and said, "You're probably wondering about what happened after that last DUI. Two years in Columbia, then out on probation. Good behavior. Can you imagine that?"

He chuckled and his eyes remained fixed on mine.

I nodded again, but didn't say anything.

"It was Reverend Stevenson," he said quietly.

"What do you mean?"

"That night EMS brought me in, after the accident. He was back in the room with me and a little girl. I remember you checking me over and taking off the cervical collar. After you left the room, he walked over to my stretcher and just stood there, looking down at me. Didn't say a word—just stood there. I closed my eyes, and all of a sudden I felt his hand on my forehead. He just kept it there, and I remember thinking how big it was, and how warm. And somehow, it felt good. He didn't say anything, just kept his hand on me for a couple of minutes. Then he was gone."

He paused, shifted a little, but didn't take his eyes off mine.

"When I was in jail, I had a lot of time to think about that night and about Reverend Stevenson. Something changed in me, and I knew things had to be different. I can't explain it, but something changed. Now here I am." His face broke into a huge smile and he patted the front of his jacket. "Can you imagine that?"

Toby Bridges turned and walked out of the department.

It was hard to believe, but I *could* imagine that.

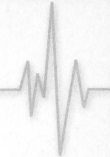

My Place

"This little girl looks pretty sick."

Lori slid the chart of room 2 in front of me and pointed to a note in the space marked "Medications."

Meds for HIV.

"Are you sure?" I glanced at the chart. The child was only five years old—young for this diagnosis.

Lori nodded. "According to her mother, she's doing great, up until a few days ago. She was exposed to the flu a week ago and now has fever and cough. Respirations are thirty and her lungs are congested."

"Thanks." I picked up the clipboard and scanned the front sheet.

Autumn Wells. 5 yr old F. Cough, fever, pneumonia.

Autumn's mother had provided this information to the secretary. If she was right about the pneumonia, that could be a real problem in a child with HIV.

The curtain of room 2 slid to one side and I stepped in, pulling it closed behind me.

"Autumn, I'm Dr. Lesslie."

She was sitting alone on the stretcher, wearing a tiny hospital gown and struggling for breath. She looked up at me with huge, brown eyes. A beautiful smile spread across her face, which was framed by curly, auburn hair. Autumn was one of those children who instantly capture your heart.

She glanced to the corner of the room and my eyes followed.

A young woman—I assumed her mother—was sitting in a chair. In her lap was another little girl who looked to be the same age as Autumn, but maybe a little younger. She was beautiful as well, but with blue eyes and blond hair. She smiled at me, then tucked her head against her mother's shoulder.

"This is Summer," the woman said. "She's a little shy."

"Hmm…" I looked back at the girl on the stretcher and again to the child in the woman's lap. "Autumn, Summer…"

"I know," the mother said. "And my name is Dakota. Dakota Wells."

"Interesting names." I put Autumn's clipboard on the stretcher, took the stethoscope from around my neck, and sat down beside the sick child.

"My father was a ranch hand in North Dakota—that's how I got my name. Just glad my parents weren't living in Idaho."

I chuckled and gently stroked the little girl's hair.

"Tell me about Autumn. When did she start getting sick?"

Dakota repeated what she had told Lori. Autumn had come down with what appeared to be a mild case of the flu, but a day or so ago it had become something worse. She was spiking temps up to 104 and her cough was getting deeper.

"She didn't sleep at all last night," her mother explained. "And we were getting worried. Then today, with the shortness of breath…Her pediatrician couldn't see her until tomorrow, so we decided to bring her here."

I finished my exam and made some notes on her chart.

"We'll need to get a chest X-ray and some blood work, but I think you're right, Ms. Wells. It looks like Autumn has pneumonia. She'll need to come in the hospital, considering how hard she's working to breathe and that she has HIV. That's going to put her at—"

"At more risk of complications," she interrupted. "I know. That's another reason why we're here. But she's done fine with her medications and has never had any problems. She's never had to be in the hospital."

I stood up and looked at the little girl. "Let's just hope it's a routine pneumonia and nothing more. But whatever it is, we'll make sure she gets better."

Autumn looked up and flashed another smile at me.

I had one hand on the curtain and was about to pull it open when I stopped and turned around.

"Tell me about Autumn and Summer—about their names."

The little blond looked up at the sound of her name and glanced at me then her mother. This time she didn't tuck her head.

"When my husband and I were first married, we tried for a couple of years to get pregnant," Dakota answered quietly. "There were several miscarriages and—we even had our nursery furnished and a name picked out. We were going to call her 'Spring.'"

Summer, Autumn, Spring. I should have guessed.

"What if it was a boy?"

Dakota shook her head and smiled. "It was *always* going to be a girl. But it didn't happen. After a few more years we gave up and decided to adopt. That's when the Lord blessed us with Autumn."

She paused and nodded at the little girl.

"We were living in Baltimore and learned about this service—or agency—for adopting children with…problems."

The HIV.

I had been struggling with the source of Autumn's infection, trying to figure out where it had come from. A child her age could have contracted it from a blood transfusion, but she had always been healthy, and there was no history of that. The other and much more likely source was from her infected birth mother.

The little girl in Dakota's lap squirmed in her mother's arms and I looked down. My hands clutched the chart I held, and I felt my face flame to a burning crimson.

Dakota looked at me, tilted her head, and her eyes followed my stare.

Her forearms were bare and I could clearly see the scars of needle tracks extending to both elbows.

She didn't flinch or try to hide them. Her eyes met mine and she smiled.

"You're right. I've had my own troubles, but those days are long past. Thankfully I don't have HIV or hepatitis, and I know I'm fortunate. Not like Autumn's…" She stopped and looked over at the stretcher. "Or Summer's," she whispered. "She's positive too."

I slumped into an empty chair and cradled the girl's clipboard against my chest. This was a lot for me to handle—something I didn't expect—something I had never experienced.

Dakota gently smoothed her daughter's golden hair and our eyes met.

"She's fine too. Never had any problems. We make sure they get the best medication possible and keep a close watch on them. But they're completely normal, and happy. That's the main thing. They're happy."

Autumn's X-ray did reveal a right-sided pneumonia. But it had all the appearances of being something routine—not what you would expect with a person with active HIV. That was good news. She would still need to be admitted but probably for only a few days.

"She's going to be fine," I told her mother.

We talked about what to expect with Autumn's treatment, and I asked Dakota when her husband would be coming to the hospital. If he was anything like his wife—and I was sure he must be—he was someone I wanted to meet.

"Dylan won't be able to get here till later. He won't get off work until after eight."

"I'll check on Autumn in the morning. Maybe I'll get the chance to meet your husband."

My hand was on the curtain again.

"Tell Miss B I said hello."

The words stunned me, and I froze.

How did Dakota know "Miss B"—my wife, Barbara? Only the little children in her classes at church knew her by that name—and the special-needs campers at Camp Joy. Where had she...?

I turned and looked at her—a giant question mark painted on my face.

Dakota smiled and nodded.

"I was in her 'Teens Under Fire' program years ago—maybe seventeen or eighteen. She might remember my name—or the goofy, belligerent teenager who sat in the back of the room staring at the ceiling and chomping on chewing gum. I don't know, though—there were probably lots of us like that."

"Teens Under Fire"—TUF—was a program my wife had put together years ago and run for more than a decade. She'd been led to reach out to the troubled youth in our community and expose them to the realities of bad decisions—violence, substance abuse and addiction, prison, and sometimes death. It was a sobering afternoon for hundreds of teenagers, most on the verge of real trouble—some already there.

"I was one of those kids in *real* trouble." Dakota shook her head and looked down at Summer. "I was making all the bad decisions Miss B was talking about. And I kept making them."

She paused and looked down at her elbows.

"I was in Tennessee when I hit rock bottom. Knoxville, in jail—headed for something worse. One night, for some reason, I started thinking about your wife—Miss B—and some of the things she'd shared with us. The main thing I remembered was that she cared—really *cared*—about us in that room. Why else would she be spending her time that way? When I woke up the next morning, I was still thinking about her and about that program, Teens Under Fire. I think I had been 'under fire' all my life and hadn't known it. That's when things started to change. I got out on probation, met Dylan, and my life has been a different journey ever since."

She gave Summer a smothering hug.

"I remember Miss B saying God only made one of us—one of *me*. And that he had a job for me in this world that no one else could do, and a place for me that no one else could fill. Back then, those were just words—but I remembered."

Dakota looked down at her daughter and then into my eyes.

"Tell Miss B I've found my place."

Still other seed fell on good soil.

Miracles OF
DELIVERANCE

*I sought the L*ORD*, and he answered me;*
He delivered me from all my fears.

PSALM 34:4

You are my hiding place;
you will protect me from trouble
and surround me with songs of deliverance.

PSALM 32:7

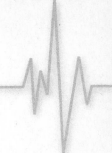

On Holy Ground

Right upper-quadrant pain—weight loss—nausea—anemia.

John Richmond was lying on the stretcher looking up at me, his eyes asking for an answer, something he could deal with. I didn't have one yet, but my gut told me that when I did, it wasn't going to be anything good.

He was sixty-six years old, a retired banker, and had always been in good health. The abdominal pain had started a few weeks earlier, but it would come and go, and he put off getting it checked out. This morning he had nearly blacked out when he got up from his kitchen chair, and that was enough for his wife, Ellen. She had insisted on his coming to the ER, and here he was.

"We need to check on some more lab work, and I'm going to get an ultrasound of your gall bladder. It might be something as simple as that." I picked up his chart and headed for the curtained entrance of room 4.

"Would that explain his anemia and almost passing out at home?" Ellen's brow furrowed and her eyes narrowed, locking on mine. She must sense something bad was going on here.

I turned and held the clipboard to my chest. "Not necessarily, but let's start there. We need to find out what's causing all of this, and I'm not going to let your husband go home until we do."

Her face softened and she smiled and nodded at her husband. I glanced down. Her hand still gripped the stretcher rail, her knuckles white and tense.

There were some troubling findings on the ultrasound, and the radiologist recommended a CT scan. That, along with the rest of his labs, confirmed the diagnosis and my worst fears. John Richmond had a large tumor in his colon and multiple metastases in his liver. There was not going to be an easy answer.

The Richmonds' son Matthew had joined them in room 4, and I shook his hand before pulling up a stool and sitting down.

"John, Ellen—we need to talk about what we've found."

His surgeon was able to remove the cancer in his colon. But the tumors in his liver didn't respond to chemotherapy and continued to grow. Within a few months he was jaundiced, his skin turning a deep yellow because of the inability of his liver to function properly. And the pain was getting worse. That was what usually brought him to the ER—and episodes of severe and uncontrollable vomiting.

"We'll get you something for the nausea in just a minute, Mr. Richmond, and something for the pain," I overheard one of my partners, Jay Barton, tell him. He was taking care of John Richmond this morning.

A few minutes later, Jay came out of room 5, pulled the curtain behind him, and walked over to the nurses' station.

"How's he doing?" I looked up from the chart in front of me and over to Jay Barton.

"Not good." Jay shook his head and slid Richmond's chart across the counter to Amy Connors. "His jaundice is worse, and his blood pressure is low. No fever—that's at least one good thing. But I can't imagine he can go on much longer like this."

"Hmm. Is his wife in there with him?"

"No, it's his daughter—Rebecca, I think. I wanted to ask him about a living will, advanced directives, that sort of thing. But I felt awkward with his daughter there and all. I wonder if he's thought about that."

"Got 'em right here." Amy held up a sheaf of papers. "He filled these out a couple of months ago and gave us a copy. Keep 'em here with his chart all the time."

She put the forms back with the rest of his record.

"Well, that's good." Jay sighed and picked up the chart for his next patient in the ENT room. "Let's see what we've got back there."

He disappeared down the hallway, and Rebecca stepped out of room 5 and walked over beside me.

"Dr. Lesslie, I'm going out to the waiting room to make some phone calls. Dad would like to speak to you, if you have a moment."

"Sure, I'll do that right now."

She didn't move, just kept looking at me with reddened eyes. Her mouth opened, but there was only a quiet sigh. She turned and walked out through triage.

"John, your daughter said you wanted to see me." I pulled the curtain closed and stepped over to his stretcher. He held out his hand—cool, damp, his handshake weak. Just that small amount of effort seemed to tire him.

"Thanks, Dr. Lesslie." His words were mumbled, whispered, and I leaned closer.

"I want to talk with you about my living will, in case...*when* something happens. I'm worried about my wife and my children. You know what they've had to go through, with all the treatments and everything."

He paused and took some deep breaths. *Worried about his wife and children.* I marveled at the strength of this man. He was dying, yet he was more concerned about his family than himself.

"I'm ready," he continued. "And I'd like nothing better than to take my last breath at home, in my bed, with my family around me. But I'm not sure...when the time *does* come...if they'll be able to..." His words drifted away. His eyes never left mine and for a moment we were both silent.

"John, I understand. And if your wife needs to have you brought here, that will be fine. We'll take care of you. And we'll take care of her."

Tears welled in his eyes, his voice just barely a whisper. "Thanks, Doctor. I just worry that Ellen..."

"It's okay, John. When the time comes, it will be okay."

Two weeks passed, and the time came. Ellen Richmond called 9-1-1 when John's breathing became labored and he started weaving in and out of consciousness. Lori Davidson directed the paramedics to the cardiac room, then walked over beside me.

"Denton Roberts said there's a bunch of people out in the waiting room, and they all want to come back. I'm sure it's his family."

I glanced over at the cardiac door and then at Lori.

"His wife handed me his advanced directives—no code—just supportive measures." She paused and shook her head. "I can't believe he can live more than an hour or so."

Lori had spent a lot of years in the ER with a lot of sick and dying patients. She knew what she was talking about.

"Sure. Let them come back."

She nodded and walked out to the waiting room.

"This is what we need on the man over in 1." I slid the chart across the counter to Amy. "See if you can get the X-ray done first."

The door of cardiac opened behind me and I turned to see Lori stepping into the hallway. She left the door cracked, looked over at me, and nodded. I had asked her to let me know when she had Mr. Richmond settled and as comfortable as we could make him.

She walked behind the nurses' station and slumped into a chair beside Amy.

The door creaked faintly as I pulled it closed behind me and stepped into the room. No one looked up.

They were all there. Ellen stood at the head of the stretcher, one hand on John's chest. Around the bed were his children—Matthew, Rebecca, and another son, Luke. With them were their spouses, and they all held hands.

If anyone was sobbing, I didn't hear it. Their heads were bowed, and the only sound in the room was the quiet, irregular breathing of John Richmond.

It was his son Matthew who began to pray, his words measured, peaceful—words of hope and faith and love. And words of thanksgiving for this man, forever delivered from his pain and suffering. Then there was John's last breath—a final *amen*.

We were silent. I knew we were standing on holy ground.

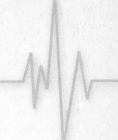

To Have and to Hold

Lori Davidson closed the curtain of room 4 and walked over to the nurses' station.

"What's the matter?" Amy Connors had twisted around in her chair and was looking up at the nurse. I glanced at her too, and saw the troubled look on her face.

Lori put an index finger to her pursed lips and shook her head. Once she was in the chair beside Amy and had put the chart of room 4 on the counter, she leaned close to the secretary and said, "This woman is in trouble." She tapped the clipboard quietly and again shook her head.

Amy shifted in her chair, straining to read the information on the chart.

"'Stephanie Evans, forty-two-year-old female. Headache and chest pain.' Is she having a heart attack?" Amy looked up at the nurse and reached for her telephone.

"No, she's not having a heart attack." Lori's voice was flat, distant. "She's not even having any chest pain."

This was unusual behavior for the nurse. I reached over the counter and she handed me the chart.

Vital signs were fine. No fever or rapid heart rate. I didn't see any red flags on the info sheet.

Lori quietly stood, caught my eye, and motioned with her head to the medicine room. I followed her across the hall, the clipboard of room 4 still in my hand. She stood near the window, gazing out onto the ER parking lot. When she turned around, there were tears in her eyes.

"Sometimes it all comes back, and I...have a hard time handling it."

I looked around for some Kleenex, couldn't find any, and handed her some dressing gauze—and waited.

"You remember my sister, don't you?" She dabbed at her eyes and sniffed.

"Angie? Sure, I remember her." Lori had brought her sister to one of our Christmas parties a few years ago. "Does she still live in Charleston?"

"No, she left Charleston last summer and moved in with our parents in Virginia. She and her two children."

That was odd. She was married, and Lori would have told us had anything happened to her sister's husband.

"What about—"

"Angie left her husband. Finally." Her face flushed and she tossed the gauze into a nearby trash can. "Finally."

I leaned back against the counter and studied her knitted brow and narrowed eyes. This was the angriest I had ever seen her.

"Her husband beat her." The words burst from her lips. "And she just took it. It went on for months before we knew about it. But she couldn't hide a fractured cheekbone. When our father found out, I thought he was going to kill him. But it was textbook. Angie blamed herself, said she must have done something to deserve it. Angie of all people! She was a basketball and track star in high school, missed being valedictorian by half a point, and she was homecoming queen. She never had an issue with self-esteem. But when it came to this...I didn't understand. None of us did."

She sighed and stared down at the floor, silent.

After a moment, I asked, "What was the breaking point? What made her leave him?"

Lori looked at me, her eyes misting again. "He hurt one of the children—twisted Jake's arm and almost broke it. Angie was in the car with the kids and on the road before her husband could turn around."

"And you think..." I held up Stephanie Evans's chart.

"Her husband is abusing her." Lori's words were measured, convicted. "I looked for an opportunity to ask her about it, but she kept deflecting me, changing the subject. You'll see when you talk with her. You'll know. You might want to ask her why she's wearing a turtlenecked sweater in the middle of summer."

All of the warning signs were there. Stephanie Evans never made eye contact with me. Her complaints were vague and ever-changing. Her answers to my direct questions were evasive, confused. There was no apparent reason for her being in the ER, except that beneath this façade, Stephanie knew she needed help. She just didn't know how to ask for it.

"How did this happen?" As part of my exam, I was checking her thyroid gland and anterior neck. Lori was right. Why would she be wearing a turtlenecked sweater when it was ninety degrees outside? I had rolled it down and saw the bruises. They were clearly in the shape of fingers encircling her throat and were of different stages of resolution. This had been going on for a while.

"What are you talking about?" Stephanie's hands flew to her neck and she pulled the sweater up to her chin.

"These bruises look like someone has choked you, Mrs. Evans. Is that how it happened?"

"I…I don't know what you mean."

Her eyes darted around the room, and then found mine. Her face softened and her lips parted, trembling. Maybe…

She turned her head and stared at the floor.

"We have a big dog, and she must have…She likes to jump up on people and she…A couple of days ago she—"

"Mrs. Evans, these bruises were made by someone's fingers."

My hand was on her collar again and she moved away, twisting on the stretcher and placing both hands around her neck.

"It was my dog."

"Mrs. Evans—"

"It was my dog."

The window slammed shut and my opportunity was gone. *What could I do? What more could I say?*

I had been in this situation more than once. We had patients who we were sure were being abused, and when we offered our help, it was rejected. Denial and fear are powerful emotions.

Many times we called the police anyway, concerned for our patients' very lives. But they were powerless to intervene unless the victim complained. When met by silence, the officers would shake their heads, give them a card with their name and phone number should they change their minds, and walk out of the department. They knew, as we did, that this wouldn't go away. It wouldn't stop. Several episodes of choking were clear evidence of the anger and intent of Stephanie's husband. It was only a matter of time.

"Mrs. Evans."

Silence.

"Any luck?" Amy Connors looked over the counter at me as I came up beside Lori. "Was she willing to talk about it?" The nurse had told her what was going on and that we might need to make a call to the police.

"She won't talk about it." I dropped the clipboard on the countertop. "I tried, but she just won't talk. But you're right, Lori. That woman is in trouble. She needs some help."

"I just don't get it," Amy muttered. "If that was me— Wait a minute! That explains it!"

She opened one of the drawers beneath the counter and flipped through a large folder of ER records from the past thirty days.

"Here it is." She slammed the drawer shut and held up the copy of an info sheet. "Stephanie Evans was in the ER a couple of weeks ago. You guys weren't here that day, and she saw Dr. Given. She said she had fallen in the bathroom and her X-rays showed two broken ribs. I remember Dr. Given sayin' things didn't add up, with what she was sayin' and what he was seein'. But she stuck to her story, and he sent her home."

Lori and I looked at each other.

"I'm going to talk with her again." She was standing behind Amy and turned in the direction of room 4. "I'm going to tell her about Angie."

Fifteen long minutes later, Lori Davidson walked back up to the nurses' station. Her eyes were reddened and her face flushed.

"Amy, would you call the police. We need them in room 4."

From this day forward...

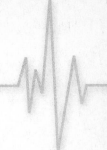

The Locusts

"Hey, Dave," I called out to the tall, trim, sixty-year-old police officer. "What brings you to the ER this morning?"

Dave Hawkins was walking through the ambulance entrance. He looked over, smiled, and gave me a mock salute. Beside him walked another policeman—one I didn't recognize. They walked over to the nurses' station and Hawkins shook my hand.

"We've got a couple of people from a fender bender in the waiting room. Nothing serious. Just want to get the investigation done and the paperwork finished." He turned to the officer beside him. "This is Private Tim Painter, my new partner. First week on the job and I'm showing him the ropes."

Virginia Granger appeared in the doorway of the medicine room. "You've got a good teacher, Officer Painter," she called out. "Just pay attention to Dave and you'll do just fine."

Lori Davidson walked through the triage entrance, leading three slouching teenage boys. When they saw the officers, their heads suddenly ducked and turned away.

"These mine?" Dave asked the nurse.

"Yep," Lori answered. "Apparently pulled out of the Burger King without looking. I'm taking them back to minor trauma."

Hawkins and Painter started off behind them. "Good," Dave said. "We'll get our part done as fast as we can. Don't want them to be late for school."

He winked and gave me another salute.

Virginia sat down behind the counter and passed a notebook to Amy Connors. "These are last month's admissions."

Amy nodded, opened a large drawer, and filed it away.

"We just get busier every month." The head nurse shook her head and looked up at me. "I'm not sure we can see many more people."

She was right, but I was more interested in Dave Hawkins.

"What do you know about Officer Hawkins? Is he a sergeant or captain? He's been around since we've been in Rock Hill, and that must be almost twenty years."

"Let's see," Amy mused, looking up at the ceiling. "You started here right after the American Revolution, so that would be—"

"Almost twenty years," I repeated, glaring at the secretary. "Not long before you. Anyway, why is he doing the same thing now as he was then? He seems like the most experienced and levelheaded officer on the force."

"You're right about that, Dr. Lesslie." Virginia nodded. "He's the best I've ever been around. He's solid and dependable, and he can calm down a volatile situation quicker than anyone I know. But he's not a sergeant or lieutenant or captain. I think he's a corporal or something like that. Something just above a private."

I glanced down the empty hallway, toward minor trauma.

"Why hasn't he advanced, or been promoted?"

Virginia shook her head. "He's had plenty of chances, and turned them down every time. He once told me he was doing what he needed to do, to be on the street and to try to make a difference. He said he had a lot to make up and didn't want to waste any more time."

"Waste more time?" I was confused. "Waste time doing what?"

Virginia looked straight into my eyes and never blinked.

"Hating."

Gary Spielman was a local hero. A track and football star at Rock Hill High, he had survived two stints in Vietnam and come home with a Purple Heart and a Silver Star. He wouldn't talk about the time he'd spent halfway around the world, but the word was he'd saved his platoon of fourteen men, putting himself at risk and receiving several pieces of shrapnel in return.

It seemed only natural that Gary join the police force when he returned to Rock Hill. He was immediately paired with Dave Hawkins, a young and promising officer who had been on the force a year or two. The two quickly bonded, becoming friends as well as partners. It wasn't long before they were receiving some of the toughest assignments in the city.

The challenge for Dave was to rein in the impulsiveness of the younger officer. While in Vietnam, Gary had been the first to volunteer for dangerous tasks, frequently taking the point on perilous patrols.

"Somebody's got to be out there," he would say. "Might as well be me."

He had the same attitude on the police force, and was soon known as the go-to guy. Gary wasn't foolish or careless, though. He was *capable*, and soon had the respect of the entire department.

Hawkins and Spielman had received their assignment for the day and were almost at their patrol car.

"Hold on a minute, Dave," Sergeant Travers called out, hurrying to catch up to the two men. "I need to give you a heads-up. You're going to be in the Collier neighborhood today and you need to know that T. Gaither is operating somewhere over there."

Gary looked at his partner and tilted his head.

"Dave can tell you about Gaither," Travers said, looking at the younger man. "He's bad news, and you guys need to be careful. Just a heads-up."

Tyler Mathew Gaither—"T."—was well known to the police departments of York and several surrounding counties. If drugs were in the area—cocaine, heroin, PCP, marijuana—that's where you would find him. And violence wouldn't be far behind. He was always armed and always dangerous.

"Sounds like my kind of guy," Gary chuckled, scanning the street from the passenger seat of the patrol car.

"Possible disturbance at 302 Blanton Street. Any available unit respond."

Spielman grabbed the radio and glanced at his partner.

"We're close, right?"

Dave nodded, slowed the vehicle, and signaled a right turn. "Two minutes."

Gary pressed the send button on the radio. "Unit 14 responding."

He dropped the radio to the console, put his hand on his holstered service weapon, and said, "I wonder what this will be."

"We'll see. 'Possible disturbance'—could be anything."

Dave flipped on his lights and siren and turned onto Blanton Street. "302, right?"

"That's right," Spielman answered, leaning forward and unfastening his seat belt. "Look, Dave—over there!"

Two men were bolting down the front steps of a small brick house. They glanced over their shoulders at the approaching patrol car and disappeared through a hedge of bushes on the far side of the yard.

"That's the place," Dave said, pulling into the driveway and cutting off the motor. "I'll call for backup."

Gary was already out of the car and heading for the house, weapon drawn.

Dave looked at the radio and then his partner. "Doggone it," he muttered and jammed the radio into the holder on his leather belt.

He jumped out and hollered at Spielman. "I'm going around back. Give me two minutes before you go in."

Gary kept his eyes trained on the front door. He crouched low to the ground and waved without a word to Hawkins. He was on the porch before Dave could get to the side of the house.

Hawkins heard the slam of the closing screen door. "Doggone it."

Two muted *thumps* from inside the house—gunshots—and Hawkins was racing back to the front of the house.

He grabbed his radio and almost dropped it. "This is unit 14—shots fired—repeat—shots fired. We need backup!"

Hawkins took the steps two at a time and burst into the living room, his weapon ready to fire.

"Gary!"

The older officer took a few cautious steps into the cluttered space. There was the crash of breaking glass from the back of the house, and he froze.

"Gary!"

"Over here, Dave."

Spielman's voice was faint, weak. It had come from somewhere in a hallway leading from the back of the living room.

Hawkins glanced around the room and moved slowly, carefully toward his partner.

"Over here, Dave." Weaker this time.

Gary Spielman sat propped against a wall at the end of the hall. His unmoving arms and legs were awkwardly spread on the floor, his weapon lying a few inches from is right hand.

"Sorry, Dave. He had a kid in his arms and I couldn't…"

Hawkins rushed to his partner and knelt beside him. Two crimson stains on the front of his shirt slowly expanded then melted together, stealing the young man's life.

A whimper somewhere off to his right, and Dave was pointing his gun, ready to fire.

"The kid." Gary's voice was barely audible.

Hawkins peered into a far corner. Huddled against the wall, clutching his knees to his chest, was a three-year-old curly-headed boy. His large, tear-filled eyes stared at the officer.

"It's the kid."

Dave sat down beside his partner and put his arms around him.

"Hold on, Gary. Hold on."

Spielman's head slumped against his friend's chest, and he was gone.

T. Gaither showed up in the ER of a neighboring city with suspicious lacerations of his hands and forearms. The back door of 302 Blanton Street had been boarded shut and he had crashed through a window making his escape. He was being sutured when the police arrived and surrounded his stretcher. He never asked about his son, the child he had left behind that morning.

—᙭᙭᙭—

"From the moment Gary Spielman died in his arms, Dave was a different man." Virginia shifted in her chair, removed her glasses, and started cleaning them with a tissue. "He was hard—not mean—but you didn't want to cross him. He was still a good policeman, one of the best. But no one wanted to be his partner. I knew Chief Green back then, and we would talk about Dave once in a while. Green wanted to promote him, get him off the street. But every time that came up, Dave refused. He said he 'needed to be on the street.' It was almost as if he was looking for something or someone. There was an edge about him—a hardness born of anger and hate—and he was miserable."

"I don't see that now, Virginia. He seems to be at peace with himself. Or maybe he just does a good job hiding it."

"No," she quickly responded. "He *is* at peace now. It took ten years, but he's at peace. I'll tell you how it happened."

mm

T. Gaither was tried, found guilty of murder, and sentenced to life without chance of parole. He was in Columbia and was hardly the model inmate.

No one knows exactly how he was able to do it, but ten years into his sentence, Gaither escaped.

For seven days, he eluded the massive multistate manhunt. The focus of this search had initially been Rock Hill—his home and the location of individuals who might offer him assistance. But there was no sign of him, and the street was quiet.

Then it broke. An anonymous tip—a 4 a.m. telephone call on a Sunday morning—sent a cruising patrol car to check out an address on the south side of town. A car manned by Dave Hawkins and his newest partner, Jerome Means.

They drove slowly past the dark, neglected house—no lights or siren—and Dave's heart hammered in his chest. *If it was T. Gaither…*

The officers stopped two houses up the street and doubled back on foot.

"What do you think, Dave? Just another goose chase?"

Hawkins had seen the momentary flicker of a flashlight through one of the side windows, but didn't tell his partner.

"We'll see." His voice was low and thick, and he slipped his service weapon out of its holster. "You go around back and I'll take the front door. Wait for my signal."

Worn and warped boards on the front porch creaked their complaint under his heavy footsteps and Dave froze.

That was loud. Had someone heard it?

His ears strained for any sound from inside—nothing.

He moved more slowly now, more cautiously, and soon his hand rested on the loose and rusted doorknob.

A deep breath, and then another. His heart pounded in his ears.

Hawkins switched on his flashlight and burst through the door, his weapon pointed dead ahead.

The bright beam flooded the small, bare room and came to rest on a startled, dozing T. Gaither. He was sitting on the floor, leaning against the far wall. Several empty soft-drink cans were scattered around him, and an empty fast-food bag lay crumpled by his right hand—right beside his .38.

Gaither shielded his eyes with his left hand and reached for his gun with the other.

His outstretched palm was on the weapon when Dave said, "Don't do it. Stay right where you are and don't move."

The officer's hands were sweating but he stood rock-solid, staring at this man who had murdered his partner.

"That you, Hawkins?"

Gaither's voice was taunting, sing-song, and Dave took a half step toward him.

Jerome was still somewhere outside. And Gaither has his handprints and fingerprints all over his own gun. This was his chance. No one would know what happened in this room—only Dave Hawkins and...

"If you ask Dave what happened next, he'll be glad to tell you." Virginia leaned back in her chair and folded her hands in her lap. "His gun was pointed right at Gaither's head and he was ready to pull the trigger..."

Dave took a step forward and was stopped by an unseen force that was solid and undeniably real. Then plain as day he heard a voice say, "Stop." He thought it was Jerome Means, his partner. But Jerome was still outside. The only people in the room were Dave and T. Gaither.

His finger was tightening on the trigger again, when he heard the same voice. "Dave, stop." This time it was louder, right in his ear. He was staring at Gaither, sure that he had heard it too. But T. just grinned at him.

In that instant, Dave Hawkins had a decision to make. He knew he could kill T. Gaither and get away with it—he could avenge the death of Gary Spielman and satisfy his hatred of this man. Or…He stood there, his hands trembling, and he knew.

"…So Dave kicked Gaither's gun away and called for Jerome."

Virginia paused and glanced over my shoulder. Dave and his young partner were walking toward us, smiling and shaking their heads.

"T. Gaither is back in prison," Virginia said quietly. "But Dave Hawkins…he's free."

I will repay you for the years the locusts have eaten…

JOEL 2:25

ALMOST A *Miracle*

*The difference between a miracle and
something just short of one
is like the difference between lightning and a lightning bug.*

(WITH APOLOGIES TO MARK TWAIN)

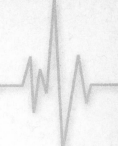

Nailed

"Rock Hill ER, this is EMS 3."

"Go ahead. This is the ER." Lori stood by the receiver, pen in hand. Amy Connors spun around in her chair and cocked her head, listening.

"We're ten minutes out with a construction injury. Twenty-nine-year-old male, nail gun to his right foot, times four."

"Four?" Amy repeated. "What th—"

"Arghh!"

The scream was loud and caused Lori to jump back from the receiver. The paramedic must be standing right beside the injured party.

"Hold on, sir, we're trying to get you some help." It sounded like Denton Roberts, one of our lead paramedics. "You need to try and relax. We'll be at the hospital in just a minute."

"Arghh! I'm going to lose my foot! I know it! I need something for the pain!"

Denton must have covered the receiver with his hand, because the next words were muffled, unintelligible. Then he was back on the radio, clear and calm.

"Like I said, we'll be there in a couple of minutes. Four nails in his right foot, through his boot. Vital signs are stable, but I can't tell about a pulse. We can't get the boot off."

Lori looked over at me and shrugged.

"Just bring him in," I told her. "Trauma room when he gets here. And Amy, call X-ray. We'll need some portable films."

Lori relayed the information to Denton, made some notes on the pad beside the radio, and hung up the receiver.

"Now how do you suppose that happened?" Amy twisted around in her chair and looked up at me. "Four nails in his foot? Seems like he would have figured somethin' was goin' on after the first one."

Lori chuckled. "We'll just have to wait and see. There must be a good reason."

"Maybe," Amy muttered. "But whatever, he sure sounded like he was in a lot of pain."

He sounded the same way a few minutes later as he was wheeled down the hallway to trauma.

"Arghh! I need somethin' for pain! My foot!"

Amy leaned over the counter, straining to get a look at the stretcher as it sped by the nurses' station. Denton wasn't wasting any time.

"Come on in here." Lori stood in the doorway to trauma, pressed against the jamb to allow them to pass.

Earl Smothers was writhing on his stretcher, desperately clutching the rails that were pulled up on each side. He was careful not to move his right foot and kept glancing down at it.

"Doc, I need something for the pain!" His eyes quickly surveyed the room and returned to his right foot. "Am I gonna lose it? Am I gonna lose my foot?"

"Try to calm down, Mr. Smothers," I told him. "We're going to take care of you. Help us get you over to our stretcher, and we'll take a look."

He grabbed his right knee, clutching it as tightly as he would a brand-new hundred-dollar bill. Without much help from our patient, we were somehow able to slide him over to the trauma bed. Denton had started an IV, and Lori quickly moved the bag of normal saline to one of our poles.

"Wide open?" She shot me a quick glance, her hand on the flow adjuster.

"Sure. At least till we know what we're dealing with."

She moved a little to one side, and for the first time I saw Earl's right foot.

Wow! Denton was right. The heads of four nails were clearly visible, each completely sunk in his worn leather work boot.

I reached down toward his foot. Like a striking rattlesnake, his hand came up and grabbed mine.

"Don't touch it, Doc! You're gonna move it and it's gonna kill me!"

"Hold on, Mr. Smothers." Lori laid a hand on his shoulder. "Dr. Lesslie is just trying to help."

I backed off, freeing my hand from his. "It's okay, Lori. Let's get an X-ray first and see exactly what we're dealing with."

"Ready when you are." Two X-ray techs were standing in the doorway, their portable machine crouched and waiting behind them.

"Good. Just get a couple of views, the best you can without moving his foot." I stepped out of their way and leaned against one of the counters.

A few minutes later, the techs were on the way back to their department, cassettes in hand. The X-rays would be developed pretty quickly.

"Earl, tell me, how did this happen? How did you manage to get four nails in your foot?"

"You ever use a nail gun, Doc?"

"Yes, I—"

"Then you know how they can have a hair trigger. *Bam bam bam bam!* It happened just like that! Four nails in my foot before I could move my finger!"

Denton Roberts was still in the room, standing near the doorway. I glanced at him, caught his eye, and he shook his head.

"Just that fast?" I was about to reach down to his foot again, but thought better of it and stopped.

"Just like that, Doc. *Bam bam bam bam!*"

The door opened and one of the X-ray techs walked in. She turned to the view box and slipped one of the films in place, then flipped on the light.

"Is that my foot, Doc?"

"It is, Mr. Smothers." I walked over to the view box and leaned close. Denton was right behind me, peering over one shoulder, with Lori hanging over the other.

There before us was his right foot, the outline of his work boot barely visible. Clearly visible, though, were the four nails, unevenly spaced and irregularly angled. They were penetrating his forefoot, the area of his toes and metatarsals.

I looked closely, trying to find any evidence of a fracture. Somehow, with injuries like this or with knives, the bones seem to slide out of the way and avoid being struck and broken. I couldn't find any evidence of a break.

Lori handed me the other film and I took the first one down. Same thing—four nails in his foot, but no visible fracture.

"Hmm, hmm."

"What's the matter, Doc? Am I gonna lose my foot?"

Earl was straining to see the view box, still grabbing his right knee to keep his foot from moving.

"I don't think so, but we need to get that boot off and take a look."

"Arghh! That's gonna kill me!"

"We'll give you something for pain first." I looked over at Lori. "How about some morphine. Start with five milligrams IV and we'll titrate it till we get some relief."

A few minutes and ten milligrams later, Earl was resting quietly on the stretcher. His hands were folded across his chest now, and he looked sleepily up at me and said, "It's okay, Doc. Do what you gotta do."

I looked over at Lori, raised my eyebrows, and shrugged. How were we going to get his boot off? We could unlace it, but the nails were stuck in his foot and we couldn't slide it off. We would have to *cut* it off.

Lori turned around and began rummaging through one of the drawers under the counter. She pulled something out, turned to me, and held it up—a pair of bandage scissors. Flimsy at best, and I shook my head.

"Ahem."

We both looked over to the corner of the room. Denton leaned casually against the wall. He slowly stood upright, reached into his back pocket, and took out a gigantic pair of scissors—more like pruning shears.

"We use these when we need to cut someone loose," he drawled.

"Perfect. Bring them over here."

I made room for him beside me at the stretcher, and began to carefully unlace Earl's work boot. Sawdust freed from the cuff of his blue jeans scattered over the bed. His eyes didn't open and he didn't move.

"Keep the morphine handy," I whispered to Lori. She held up a loaded syringe and waved it at me.

I loosened the top of the boot as much as possible, then motioned for Denton to start cutting. Together, with me holding leather and him carefully snipping, we began to remove his boot, one piece at a time.

The work went faster than I thought possible, and we soon reached the first nail. No blood, or at least none visible on the top of his foot.

"Hasn't washed these socks in a while," the paramedic whispered, frowning and wrinkling his nose.

I nodded and gingerly took hold of the top of the nail. Once freed from the boot, it was loose, and moved easily. Denton trimmed the odiferous sock away, and our eyes widened. The nail was snuggled up against Earl's great toe, but there was no blood. It hadn't penetrated the skin.

We kept working, trimming the leather away from the next nail. The sock fell away, and we stared at each other. The nail had passed cleanly between the great and second toes, but again, there was no blood and no broken skin.

The third nail was the same—neatly wedged between two toes, having missed his foot entirely.

Lori shook her head, looked down at the sleeping Earl, and then at the morphine-filled syringe. Without a word, she turned and set it on the countertop.

The last nail was different. We freed it from leather and cotton, but it wouldn't move. It was stuck firmly. This must be the one that was causing his pain.

Denton trimmed some more of the boot away and I leaned down, my face almost touching the stretcher.

There it was. I let out a loud sigh and shook my head. The nail was jammed in the bottom of his boot, slap up against his little toe. And here was the blood. Actually, it was a drop at most, just a little scratch. Somehow all four nails had missed his foot and toes.

Earl shifted on the stretcher, and his head rolled to one side and then lazily up to where he could see us.

"Doc, am I gonna lose my foot?"

"No, Earl—you're going to be alright."

His head flopped back down onto the stretcher.

"Well, thank the Lord."

All Swole Up

"Dr. Lesslie, do you remember me?"

I was standing in line in the grocery store and the question caused me to tense, just like it always did.

The words had come from behind me and I slowly turned and stood face-to-face with a middle-aged woman. She was smiling. Yes! It was going to be something good.

She looked familiar, but I couldn't quite place her. And I for sure couldn't remember her name. That's one skill I haven't mastered—remembering names. Just ask my wife. *Her* name is...dang it! It'll come to me.

"You saw my little girl in the ER about eight or nine years ago." The woman was beaming now, and her eyes were dancing. "I'm just so glad I bumped into you. All these years, and I've been wanting to thank you."

I waited, still not remembering this woman or her daughter.

She patted the head of the girl standing beside her. "Nobody could figure out what was wrong with Adele. Not until we came and saw you that night in the ER."

It was my turn, and I had to say *something*. "I'm glad she's better." *How lame was that?*

"Better? She's *better* than better. She's fine now. But for a couple of weeks there, we were really worried, what with her legs swelling up all the time. Could barely walk."

It was starting to come back now, and I looked more closely at the woman's face. Her daughter would have been a teenager eight or nine years ago—and with swollen legs that were bad enough to bring her to the ER. Then I remembered.

Jay Barton had been working the morning shift with me. He had finished his emergency-medicine residency a couple of years earlier. Jay knew his stuff, but the thirteen-year-old girl he was seeing in room 2 had him stumped.

We stood beside each other at the nurses' station, and I watched as he drummed the girl's record with the fingers of his right hand.

"This just doesn't make sense." He stopped his drumming and loudly slapped the chart. "Perfectly healthy up until a few weeks ago, then started having some swelling in her legs, mainly in the morning. It's bad enough to keep her from putting on her shoes. Gets better during the day, when she's up on her feet, and starts all over again the next morning."

I glanced down at the girl's record.

Adele Hoskins. Legs swole up.

"Descriptive." I pointed at the word *swole*.

"The secretaries up front just type what the patient says. Or in this case, the mother. But it *is* descriptive. She *is* all swole up."

He chuckled but then scratched his chin and frowned.

"Vital signs are fine." I pointed to her blood pressure and pulse. "Any weight gain or shortness of breath?"

"No, none of that. My first thought was her kidneys—she's a little old for nephrotic syndrome, but I guess it could happen. That would explain the edema. But like you said, her blood pressure is fine, and there's no protein in her urine. I'm waiting on some lab work and a chest X-ray, but so far I'm drawing blanks. Other than the swelling, she's completely normal."

"Dr. Barton, Dr. James is on the phone." Amy Connors held the receiver over the counter and Jay grabbed it. He placed a hand over the mouthpiece and whispered, "This is her family doctor, and her mother said Adele's been in the office three or four times with this. I want to see what he—"

He put the phone to his ear. "Bradley, this is Jay Barton. Thanks for returning my call. We've got Adele Hoskins here in the ER with her legs swollen again. Any thoughts as to what might be causing this?"

I walked down the hallway to a waiting patient in the ENT room. Fifteen minutes later, Jay was still at the nurses' station. He was no longer on the phone, and still scratching his chin.

"James has no clue either," he said with a sigh. "He's ruled out heart disease and kidney problems. Thinks it might be some strange auto-immune disease, something that's just not showing up in her blood work yet. He's going to send her to Duke and see what they think about it."

"Did he have any suggestions about what you need to do for her today?" I understood his predicament and frustration. The only bright spot here was that Adele was his patient and not mine.

"No. He says he's looked under every rock he can think to look under and hasn't found a thing. He'll be glad to see her in the office, but I sense Mrs. Hoskins is not interested in going that route anymore. That's why she's here."

Jay sighed and glanced at the closed curtain of room 2. "I guess I'll go talk with her and explain what we've found. Or haven't found."

The next time I walked up to the nurses' station, the curtain of room 2 was pulled open and the room was empty.

A week later, it was my turn.

"She's back." Amy slid the chart across the counter. "Same thing. Swole legs."

I didn't have to look at the record to know the name of the patient.

Adele was in room 2 again. I pulled the curtain closed behind me and walked over to the stretcher.

Her legs were indeed "swole." From the knees down, they were both distended and tense. But there was no pain, no tenderness, and her pulses were completely normal.

"Dr. Lesslie, we need some help here." Mrs. Hoskins was pleading, wringing her hands, and pacing the small room. "It's just not getting any better."

Her heart and lung exams were normal, and I told them we would check another urine specimen, just to be sure nothing had developed since her last visit. But there was no reason to repeat another lengthy workup.

Lori Davidson led Adele to a nearby bathroom and gave her instructions for collecting a urine specimen. After that, she walked her back to room 2, pulled the curtain closed behind her, and was in there for what I thought was a long time. When Lori finally came out, she looked at me, smiled, and shook her head as she walked over.

"What is it? What's so funny?"

Lori put the full specimen cup on the counter. "We won't need to be checking her urine. It's going to be completely normal."

"How can you be so sure? How can—"

"I've made the diagnosis, Dr. Lesslie. I know what's causing the swelling in Adele's legs."

Mrs. Hoskins was standing beside Adele's stretcher, gently stroking the girl's long brown hair. She looked up as I walked into the room.

"Adele, let's go over a couple of things." I pulled a stool up and sat down, her clipboard in my lap. "Tell me about this knee pain you've been having."

The teenager's eyes widened and she looked over at her mother.

Mrs. Hoskins spoke. "She was having some pain in her knees—growing pains—that's all. Didn't fall or anything, and I told her to take some ibuprofen. That helped—didn't it, honey?"

Adele was staring at her mother. She nodded, then looked at the floor and shook her head.

I cleared my throat and shifted a little on the stool. "What have you been doing for your knee pain?" Mrs. Hoskins stopped stroking the girl's hair. She stood ramrod straight, tilted her head to one side, and stared at her daughter.

"I've been..." Adele looked up at her mother, then suddenly fell silent.

"Tell the doctor, child. What have you been doing?"

"I've been wrapping my knees up at night, right before I go to bed. I found some Ace bandages in the bathroom and I've been using those." She sighed and slumped against the wall behind her.

"Have you been putting those bandages on tight?" I knew the answer, but needed to hear it.

"As tight as I could. And it helped. The pain was gone in the morning, but my legs were all swollen."

Mrs. Hoskins stood with her hands on her hips, mouth gaping, shaking her head in silence.

"You've been doing this every night?" I placed a hand on one of her swollen ankles. The Ace bandages had acted like tourniquets. Causing fluid to collect in her legs overnight.

"Uh-huh."

I glanced over at her mother and then back down at Adele.

"Okay, here's what we're going to do."

I hadn't seen Adele or her mother in the intervening eight years and never heard what happened with the girl's "swole" legs.

"Like I said, Dr. Lesslie, Adele is fine now. Completely normal. No more swelling after that day. And it was all thanks to you. If you hadn't have figured out about those Ace bandages, who knows what would have happened."

She needed to know the truth here—that Lori Davidson had been the diagnostician. "Mrs. Hoskins, I—"

She shushed me with a waving index finger.

"Nope, none of that. I just wanted to thank you for helping Adele. It was amazing. No, it was a…"

Little Children, Fools, and Drunks

"EMS 2, respond code 3 to a 10-50, 1492 Orchard Road. Presumed PI's."

Denton Roberts and his partner, Rob Flynn, were wolfing down a couple of Wendy's cheeseburgers. Several nearby customers glanced at the squawking radio sitting on the paramedics' table. Denton picked it up and pressed a large red button.

"This is EMS 2. We'll be en route in one minute."

Rob looked at the burger in his hand, shook his head, wrapped it in a couple of napkins, and stuffed it in his jacket pocket.

"You sure about that?" Denton was already headed to the door.

"Hey, a man's gotta eat. And what's this about an auto accident with 'presumed PI's'? Either there're personal injuries or there're not."

"Beats me. I guess we'll find out."

Orchard Road was a good ten minutes out in the country, even at maximum safe speed. The ambulance's halogen headlights pierced the dark, moonless night, and its flashing blue-and-red lights bounced off trees and road signs as the paramedics sped to the accident.

Dispatch had informed them that a police unit was on its way and should arrive moments after they did.

"You think the driver left the scene?" Rob shifted in his seat and stuck his hand into his jacket pocket. "That might explain the 'presumed PI' business. What th—" He held his hand under the interior dome light. It was covered with ketchup and decorated with a few streaks of mustard and one lonely pickle to boot.

"I was a little worried about that." Denton chuckled, looking at his partner's hand. "But you know, a man's gotta eat. Right?"

"Now you listen—"

"Look, there it is—1492." Denton braked the ambulance and pointed to a mailbox on the right side of the road.

Rob wiped his hand on his pants and looked out his window. "Mighty dark out there. You see anything?"

They pulled onto a graveled driveway and the beams of their headlights found a small, one-story brick house. The front porch was screened, its door closed.

Denton rolled down his window as they slowly approached the house. He switched off the siren, its strident wail replaced by the quiet crunching of gravel beneath the ambulance's tires.

The porch lights turned on, painting the front of the house with a pale yellow hue.

"Look—over there."

Denton was pointing toward a large live oak. Its limbs spread spiderlike, almost touching the ground in places. Under one of these low-hanging boughs, lying on its side, was a late-model Ford truck. The motor was still running and one of the back wheels was uselessly spinning in the night air.

The porch door slammed and a middle-aged man walked toward them. He was barefoot, and his undersized T-shirt barely covered half of his oversized belly.

"You got here pretty quick, boys." He walked up to Denton's side of the ambulance and held out his hand. "Ernie Brakefield. This here's my place."

Rob Flynn was already out of the vehicle and sprinting toward the overturned truck.

"Any idea how this happened?" Denton opened the door, jumped down, and reached behind his seat for the emergency box.

"What? The wreck?" Ernie looked over at the truck and then out to the highway. "Best as I can figure out, the driver was going pretty fast and didn't see the curve over there." He was pointing somewhere off to the left, invisible in the pitch-black darkness. "He plowed through my yard and hit the drainage ditch. That's what must have flipped him over—probably a couple of times. Then he come to rest underneath that oak tree."

He had gracefully traced the presumed path of the truck, looping his hand in the air a few times before finally pointing to its resting place.

Denton turned and hurried over to his partner. Ernie huffed along behind them, struggling to keep up.

"Got anything?" Denton called out.

"Nothing yet." Rob's voice was coming from somewhere behind the truck, his body invisible.

"Not gonna find anything, either," Ernie got out between labored breaths.

They came to a stop beside the Ford, and Denton turned to the man. "You never saw the driver? Never saw anyone?"

"Nope. Not a soul. And I was out here one, maybe two minutes after it happened. I looked all around the truck and in the ditch. Even out in the road. Thought maybe the driver'd bailed out when he realized what was about to happen. But nothing. Not a trace. Whoever was behind the wheel just vanished."

A loud barking broke the silence of the quickly chilling nightfall. Denton looked over in the direction of the sudden noise and saw a young golden retriever sitting just inside the porch door, its tail sweeping the floor in long, graceful arcs.

"Hush up, Moses! Stop that barking." Ernie shook his head. "That dog's been all excited ever since this happened. Just keeps pacin' around the porch and barkin' his head off. About to drive me crazy."

The dog barked again, not paying attention to his master.

"Moses!" Ernie was growling at the dog, and this time he fell silent.

"Key's still in the ignition," Rob called out. "I'm gonna turn it off before something blows."

Flynn's flashlight cast powerful beams in and around the truck. No sign of any movement or any body.

"How much did you look around, Mr. Brakefield?" Denton set the heavy box on the ground and took his own flashlight from his belt.

"I walked around a good bit." Ernie waved his arm in a wide circle. "Like I said, I looked out by the road and way beyond the tree. I was thinkin' maybe the driver got thrown through the windshield, but there ain't no broken glass. Nothin's broke that I can see, except the front left headlight. That's hard to believe, considerin' all the noise this thing made as it plowed through my yard."

Moses started barking again, and pacing up and down in the porch.

"Moses, don't make me come over there!"

"Denton, come take a look." Rob was standing on the other side of the truck, his flashlight pointing into the vehicle.

Denton stepped through some tall grass and weeds and around to where his partner stood.

"What do you make of that?" Rob held his light in one hand and pointed to the side of the open passenger window with his other.

Denton stooped over, almost pressing his nose to the metal post. He reached out and rubbed something between his thumb and index finger.

"Feels like pants material to me—blue jeans. Looks like it was torn or ripped off."

"That's what I thought too." Rob leaned close, tracing the window frame with his flashlight. "But there's no blood anywhere."

Moses barked louder now, and without saying a word Ernie headed in the direction of the dog.

"Mr. Brakefield, hold on there." Denton straightened up and took off after the man.

Ernie spun around, looking into Denton's light. He blinked a couple of times and shielded his eyes with a stubby hand.

"What? What's the matter?"

"Has Moses been out in the yard since this happened?"

Ernie looked over his shoulder, then back at the paramedic. "No, I've kept him on the porch. He's young and too excited. Why?"

Rob walked up beside Denton and they looked at each other.

"Why don't we let Moses loose and see what he does?" Denton pointed his beam at the porch. "Maybe he can find something."

"Listen! What's that?" Ernie stood as still as a fence post and stared up into the night sky.

Rob cocked his head and strained his ears. The thick darkness was broken by the faint but unmistakable wail of a siren.

"Good," Rob said. "The police should be here in a few minutes."

They turned in the direction of the porch. Moses was still pacing, still barking.

"Might as well give him a try. Can't hurt anything." Ernie stumped off toward the house with Rob and Denton close behind.

They reached the porch door. The retriever was ready to explode out. He was whining now, his body a mass of wriggling muscle.

"Better back up," Ernie warned. "He don't know his own strength."

Brakefield opened the porch door and jumped out of the way. Moses bounded through the opening and straight over to the truck. He circled it once, sniffing the ground, stopped still as a statue, and held his nose in the air.

The three men watched as the dog's tail began to slowly swish.

"Look. He's got somethin'," Ernie whispered.

Moses was looking up into the tree, still sniffing the night air. His head turned to the house and he took a couple of cautious steps toward the porch.

He stopped once more, uttered a low growl, then let forth a couple of thunderous barks.

Denton and Rob jumped backward, their lights focused on the dog.

"Look, I told you he had somethin'."

Moses looked up at the roof of the house and started to pace back and forth in front of the porch.

Rob trained his flashlight on the edge of the weathered gutter and carefully followed it, starting at the right-hand corner.

The beam of light froze halfway down the porch.

"Look! Do you see that?" Rob stepped closer to this house, his light not wavering from the spot.

Denton was peering at the edge of the roof, his light joining Rob's. "It looks like a—"

"It's a foot!" Ernie hurried over to the house, pointing at the gutter. Moses was right beside him, jumping up and down and agreeing with sharp, nervous yelps.

While the three men and the dog watched, the foot twitched once, and then again. This started Moses barking even louder.

"Shh! Listen!" Denton held out his hand.

Ernie reached down and grabbed Moses by the collar. "Quiet, boy. Quiet."

"Hear that?" Denton whispered.

Six human and two canine ears strained mightily, all eyes locked on the dangling shoe.

A low moan floated down to them from the roof, and then a hand slowly came into view, waved weakly, and collapsed back into the darkness.

Denton Roberts shared this story with me two days later in the ER. He and Rob had brought in an ankle injury from a local skating rink and he had pulled me aside at the nurses' station.

"It was a twenty-eight-year-old guy who'd just left a bar over in York. Lost control of his car, flipped it a couple of times, and was thrown through the passenger window. No seat belt, of course. Landed on the roof, right where we found him. Or right where Moses found him."

"How did you get him down?" This was a crazy story, but I knew it was true. Parts of it had been in the local paper.

"That wasn't easy. The police got there, then a fire engine. We used their bucket to get him to the ground and then helicoptered him to the trauma center in Charlotte."

I stopped writing on the chart in front of me and looked over at Denton. "How's he doing now?"

"That's the darnedest thing, Doc." The paramedic put his hands on his hips and shook his head. "That guy found out where Rob and I were working and walked into the station this morning, pretty as you please. Had a couple of scratches on his arms and face, but that was it. Nothing serious. The docs in Charlotte couldn't believe he'd flown a good thirty or forty feet in the air. They thought it must have been a miracle. Either that or his blood alcohol of four times legally drunk. What's that they say about God looking after little children, fools, and drunks? Anyway, he didn't remember much of anything, except feelin' like he was flyin' and then a dog barkin'. That's one lucky guy, and he knows it. Somebody upstairs was lookin' after him that night."

Little children, fools, and drunks. Two out of three. He was *more* than lucky.

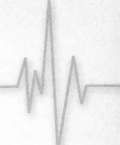

Miracle Worker

I heard and felt the *clunk* as the thirty-year-old man's dislocated shoulder slipped back into place. He had injured it while playing rugby, and Jim Given, our youngest partner, had been the first to see him.

"I've only done a couple of these, Robert, and could use your help if you have the time."

I had walked him through the procedure and steadied the man's shoulder while Jim tried several maneuvers.

Clunk—and it was done.

"Ahhhhh. That feels great."

In spite of the morphine and Versed on board, our patient had been grimacing and tightly squinting his eyes. Now they opened and he looked into the face of Jim Given.

"Thank you, Doc," he mumbled, a huge smile spreading from ear to ear. "You're a miracle worker."

"No, I'm not a miracle worker." Jim stammered and shook his head. "I'm just glad that—"

"Doc, I'm telling you—you're a *miracle* worker."

Thus are legends born.

"Thanks, Dr. Given—I know I'll feel better real soon."

Thad Summers held a prescription in his hand and waved it in the air as he walked down the hallway. He worked in the hospital's engineering department and had come by the ER to be seen, complaining of a bad case of bronchitis.

"That guy thinks you walk on water," I said to Jim Given. He was standing beside me at the nurses' station and glanced up. I nodded at Thad as he disappeared around the corner in the back of the department.

"Yeah, he says you're a real miracle worker." Amy Connors looked up from her logbook and chuckled.

"What makes you say that?" Given asked her. He was young and green enough to remember how to blush, and his face turned a light pink.

"Remember when you saw Thad a couple of months ago?" Amy cocked her head to one side. "He came down here complainin' of low-back pain. He thought it was sciatica. His doctor had ordered a scan of his back lookin' for a ruptured disc but nothin' showed up. His doc had him on a bunch of medicine but he wasn't gettin' any better."

Jim Given rested an elbow on the counter and rubbed his chin. "I'm not sure if—"

"You were standing right where you are now." Amy pointed to the floor behind him. "He walked by holdin' his back and you asked him what the problem was. He started talkin' about his back and the scan and that he wasn't gettin' any relief."

"I remember now." Given nodded his head and slapped the countertop. "He had a huge wallet in his back pocket and I told him to get rid of it, or at least move it from where it was. It was big enough to be pressing on his sacroiliac area and cause his symptoms."

"Well, you were right," Amy beamed. "He got rid of that wallet and within a week his pain was gone. He told me you were a miracle worker for sure."

Given blushed again. "I don't know about that. It just seemed obvious to me, and I—"

"What about the mother last week?" I interrupted. "The woman who came in with her three-year-old because he wouldn't move his elbow? His uncle had been slinging him around by his arms and the child started crying and wouldn't move his left arm."

"That was straightforward." Given shook his head and waved his hand at me. "Nursemaid's elbow. Any rookie would have known that."

"Not necessarily," I corrected him. "She had already seen her family doctor and he thought the arm was broken. That's why they were here—to get an X-ray. Didn't you take care of that child while he was out in triage?"

"Yeah, I did. Jeff Ryan grabbed me and took me out there and I reduced it while the boy was sitting in his mother's lap."

"We heard him holler way out here," Amy laughed. "But in a couple of minutes his mother brought him through triage and he was smilin' and wavin' at everybody—with his *bad* arm. You were already in another room, and that momma just kept on singin' your praises."

"Straightforward," Given murmured. "Like I said."

"What *wasn't* straightforward was that fifteen-year-old girl you took care of last weekend," I reminded him. "Brought in by EMS, unresponsive."

"The one who took her father's medication?" Amy leaned forward in her chair, her arms on the desktop.

"Yeah, that's the one." I looked at Given.

He stood beside me, quietly nodding. "Now *that* was difficult," he sighed. "At least until we were able to get a reliable history. Nobody knew anything, except that she was unconscious, passed out. The whole family was yelling and screaming and running around in circles. Grandma thought the girl had a stroke or something. I think it was her little brother who finally came forward and told us what happened."

"Didn't she take her father's diabetic pills?" Amy asked. "That's what I seem to remember."

"You're right, Amy," Given nodded at her. "Her little brother had gotten hold of their father's diabetic medicine and he dared her to take some. She took enough to drop her blood sugar to the point where she lost consciousness. The boy was too scared to say anything until he thought she was going to die."

Jeff Ryan had walked up to the nurses' station and heard this last story. "That's right. You ordered IV glucose and we barely touched her with it when she sat straight up on the stretcher, looked around, and started singing."

"Strangest reaction I've ever seen." Jim Given shook his head and looked down at the countertop.

"No," Jeff laughed. "The *strangest* reaction I've ever seen was when that grandmother grabbed you and started squeezing and slinging you around. Said you had saved the girl's life and that you had a special anointing, or something like that."

"Anointin'?" Amy asked. "You mean like in the Bible?"

"Listen, it was simple," Given explained, a hint of exasperation in his voice. "Once we knew the problem, it was easy to fix with some glucose. We got her blood sugar up and she—"

"And she started singing," Jeff chuckled. "And grandma started hugging and hollering. It didn't matter *how* it happened, you were the real hero that day."

Jim stood there and shook his head. "Okay, that's about enough."

He was rattled and we weren't about to let him off the hook.

"Now that you mention it, Jeff, Dr. Given *has* been the hero a lot lately. What about that twenty-year-old who took his friend's antipsychotic medication?"

"I almost forgot about that guy." The nurse leaned against the counter and rubbed his hands together. "He came through the ambulance entrance late one night with his girlfriend. She was screaming for help at the top of her lungs. It was one of the oddest things I've ever seen—the medicine was causing his hands to scrunch up and he was leaning to one side. His head was down on his chest and he couldn't talk because his tongue wouldn't work."

I looked over at Jim. His eyes were closed and he slowly shook his head. "Dystonic reaction," he muttered. "Straightforward."

"Dr. Given knew just what to do," Jeff continued. "'IV Benadryl!' he hollered. We got a line started, gave him the Benadryl, and in a couple of minutes that guy was standing up straight, talking, and heading for the door. It was *something* all right."

"What about the eighty-year-old gentleman from down in Edgemoor?" Amy was on the edge of her chair, rocking back and forth. "Said he couldn't hear a thing and needed some help. Remember him?"

"That's right!" Jeff slapped his palms on the countertop. "I almost forgot about him too. I was working triage that afternoon and put him in the ENT room. Nice guy, but he couldn't hear a thing. Dr. Given went in, examined him, and asked Lori to wash out his ears. She said she got enough stuff out to plant potatoes. But it fixed him. He could hear."

Jim Given's eyes were still closed and he sighed loudly.

"Lori said when Dr. Given went in to check him, the man jumped up and hollered 'Hallelujah!' Knocked the irrigation stand over and water went everywhere."

"Now *that* would have been an anointin'," Amy smirked.

"That's it. I've had enough."

Jim Given spun around and stomped off down the hallway.

Miracle worker.

...the difference between lightning and a lightning bug.

The *Miracle* OF ANGELS

Angels descending bring from above
Echoes of mercy, whispers of love.

FANNY CROSBY (1820–1915),
from the hymn "Blessed Assurance"

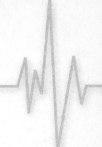

In His Care

It was a Sunday morning, and the after-church crowd was still a few hours from hitting the ER. We were quiet, with only a few patients scattered around the department.

Amy Connors logged in the next patient, slid the chart of minor trauma C across the countertop, looked up at me, and said, "Busted head, seventy-two-year-old. A little unusual for this time of day."

"Amy, you know better than that. Not much around here is unusual."

"Yeah, right. But still."

She turned in her chair, picked up a stack of charts, and starting filing them in one of the desk drawers.

I picked up the chart and scanned the "patient information" section. *Roy Littlejohn. 72-year-old male. Lacerated scalp—alleged assault.*

"Alleged assault." Now that *was* a little unusual for this time of day.

The hallway was quiet as I made my way back to minor. I heard voices as I turned into the room—and came to an abrupt stop.

On the stretcher in the back-right corner sat an elderly man, clutching a blood-soaked kitchen towel and holding it to the back of his head. He looked up at me, raised his other hand, and smiled. Mr. Littlejohn.

But who were these other people?

There were no other patients on the three remaining beds, but the room was crowded. I recognized the police officer who was there, Jimmy Bagwell. He was standing at the head of the stretcher, making notes on a small notepad. He looked over at me and raised two fingers to the front of his hat. I nodded.

Jammed behind the stretcher were two young boys, probably ten or eleven years old. They stood tensely, their arms folded across their chests with hands in their armpits. They didn't look up, and their eyes were glued on Mr. Littlejohn.

Sitting in a chair at the foot of the stretcher was an elderly woman. She wore a flowered housecoat, tattered at the edges, and her hair was covered with a purple scarf. One hand rested on the man's knee. *This must be his wife.* She looked over at me and dabbed a reddened eye with a much-used Kleenex.

Lori Davidson stood with her back to me, opening a suture kit on the countertop. She should know better. Our rooms were small, and our policy was to have only one family member with a patient. Otherwise things got crowded and sometimes out of hand.

She turned and our eyes met. I tilted my head and furrowed my brow. She just smiled, shrugged her shoulders, picked up the suture tray, and carried it over to the metal stand beside the stretcher.

She must have a reason for this. She knew this was one of my pet peeves and—

"Doctor, this is Roy Littlejohn and his wife, Ella." The metal cups clattered together as she set them on the stand. "And these are their...boys."

I nodded at the couple and stepped over to the stretcher. The two boys never looked up.

"I'm Dr. Lesslie," I said, smiling at Ella and shaking Roy's hand. His grip was warm and strong. "Tell me what happened this morning."

"We're sorry to put you to this trouble, Doctor," Roy answered. "I know you're busy, and—"

"Three guys broke into their house this morning, Doc," Jimmy Bagwell interrupted. "Tried to rob them, and busted Roy over the back of his head with a baseball bat." Jimmy's face was flushed, and he spat out the words angrily. I looked at him and then over at Lori. She shook her head and turned away.

"We've got 'em downtown, and I came with Roy and Ella to make sure they were okay."

Roy looked up at the officer. "Thanks, Jimmy. But they didn't get anything, just a cell phone that doesn't work and five dollars off the kitchen table."

Ella shook her head and patted her husband's knee.

"Tell me exactly what happened," I said, stepping closer to the man. "Did you lose consciousness? And are you hurt anywhere other than your head?"

Roy told me about the assault, how the three young men had knocked on the door asking for help, then grabbed his arms and pushed him into the kitchen.

"There was nothing we could do," Ella said quietly. "Nothing."

The two boys awkwardly shuffled their feet, their eyes darting to each other and then back down at Roy.

He hadn't lost consciousness, and there was no other sign of any trauma, just the gaping five-inch laceration on the back of his head.

"What do you think, Doctor? Just a couple of Steri-Strips?"

"No, Roy—I'm afraid it's going to take a little more than that."

Forty-five minutes and twenty-two stitches later, we had him back together.

I stood up slowly from my stool, stretched my aching back, and turned to Lori. "He'll need a tetanus booster, and I'll write something for pain." I looked at Roy and said, "Hope that wasn't too bad, Mr. Littlejohn. And I'm sorry it happened."

"You did a fine job, and I want to thank you."

Lori followed as I headed out of the room and into the hallway.

"Dr. Lesslie, I want to apologize for all of the people in the room, but—"

I stopped and looked at her. "I figured you had a reason."

"His wife needed to be back there with him. But those two boys weren't about to leave him. It just wasn't going to happen."

"Grandsons?" I was making some notes on Roy's chart and didn't look up at her.

"No, not grandsons."

There was an odd tone in her voice, something I didn't recognize. She turned and disappeared back into minor before I could say anything.

Jimmy Bagwell was standing at the nurses' station as I walked up.

"Those are good people," he nodded down the hallway. "It just burns me up what those guys did. It's gonna be hard to get the Littlejohns to press charges, though. They know them, and said they didn't want to get them into trouble."

"After what they did to him?"

"I know. But you've got to understand Roy and Ella. The only way they'll press charges is if I can convince them it's best for the guys who did this. They need to be held accountable, and to grow up."

I shook my head and started writing on Roy's chart.

"You know about them, don't you? Roy and Ella?"

I didn't, and put down my pen and turned to the officer.

"No, I don't. Tell me."

Jimmy shifted a little and leaned on the countertop. "They live over off of White Street. Been there more than forty years. As I understand it, they could never have children of their own, so they started raisin' some of the kids in the neighborhood, the ones who had trouble or whose parents..."

"Like foster parents?"

"Yes. No...well, sort of. They aren't officially foster parents, and have never taken any money for takin' these children into their home. They just provided a safe place for troubled kids until somethin' else could be done for them. Sometimes the kids would stay with them for a couple of years. And sometimes it was the only caring and...love that these children ever knew. Like those boys back there." He nodded again down the hallway.

"Those two boys? You mean—"

"Yeah, they've been livin' with them for two, maybe three years. Their father's been in prison and their mother...Well, she has a drug problem, and she disappeared one night. Haven't heard or seen anything of her since. Maybe someday..."

I nodded and studied Jimmy's face. A cloud had passed over it, and he sighed heavily.

"That must be why those boys wouldn't leave his side," I said quietly.

"Of course they wouldn't. He and Ella are like a father and mother to them. Just like they are to a lot of people in town. Like I said, they've been doin' this for more than forty years."

"Wow, I had no idea. You just never know...I mean, they must have made a big difference in a lot of lives. Who knows what would have happened to all those children, or these two boys?"

The cloud passed from Jimmy Bagwell's face. He stood up straight and smiled at me.

"Doc, I turned out okay."

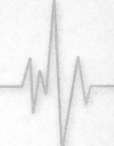

Let Slip the Dogs of War

More than one police officer has told me the most dangerous place in Rock Hill is the ER waiting room...

"Get another line going and get X-ray down here stat!"

The twenty-year-old was writhing in pain beneath my hands. He had been gut-shot with a small-caliber weapon at short range. Powder burns stippled the area around the entrance wound, just above his umbilicus. He was confused, combative—and we were losing him.

"And get lab—we need six units of blood now!"

Amy Connors was standing in the doorway, calmly making notes on a pad of paper. In spite of the chaos in the room, she wouldn't miss anything.

"Amy, where's the surgeon?"

"Still in cardiac putting in the chest tube." She kept writing and didn't look up. "They're ready in the OR as soon as they get that done."

Bill Chambers was the surgeon on call, and he was taking care of the first gunshot victim brought in by EMS. We needed help, and his partner was on the way in—none too soon for the young man in front of me.

"We gotta go, Doc." Denton Roberts was grabbing some supplies for his unit. He and his paramedic partner had brought in my patient, and they would be heading back to the scene of this violence.

"How many more out there?" I asked him. Three ambulance units had already responded, and at least two victims had been sent by helicopter to the Charlotte trauma center.

"I know they're still working three, maybe four gunshots. And there's another half-dozen walking wounded with minor knife and broken-bottle wounds. We'll bring them in last."

Three, maybe four more gunshot victims. Where were we going to put them?

Denton and his partner dashed out the door and Virginia Granger walked into the room.

"What do you need most?" As always, she was direct and to the point. I was glad to see her.

"Probably a couple of MASH units—that would be helpful."

Virginia had left for home hours ago. It was midnight, the Fourth of July, and still sweltering outside. Throw in a substantial dose of alcohol, some smoldering ill-will, and you had all the fixin's for a brawl. She had heard what was going on and had come to help.

"I'll go to triage and see if they need some assistance, and check back here in a few minutes," she volunteered.

Did I say brawl? I thought. *This is more of a war.* The principal combatant groups were the Courtney and Morrison families. Each group had some fringe gang members as well as "well-intentioned friends." The altercation had started at a local nightclub—no, that designation would be too generous. It had started in a ramshackle bar and quickly spread into the parking lot. Handguns, knives, and beer bottles were wielded to resolve any significant differences, of which there were many. It was the police department's worst nightmare, as it was for those of us who staff the ER.

Jody Bridgers had been one of the first officers to come to the department. Now he walked up behind me and put a hand on my shoulder. "I know you're busy, but it's going to get worse. I don't think I've ever seen anything like it."

I turned and looked at the sergeant. He was sweating profusely, his blue uniform plastered to his chest and arms. Sweat poured down his face and he tried unsuccessfully to stem it with a small towel.

"We might need some help here shortly, once more of the injured get here. Lori already told me the waiting room is full and getting rowdy."

Jody stuffed the towel into his pants pocket and shook his head. "I *know* you'll be needing some help *there*, but the fact is, we have every available unit at the scene. We've called in everyone we could find and still don't have enough officers. As soon as we get one group under control, another fight breaks out down the street or behind the building. It's like that game…What do you call it?"

"Whack-a-mole."

"That's right—whack-a-mole. Just like that."

The officer stepped out of the way of two lab techs. They hurried to the side of the stretcher and prepared to fill several rubber-stoppered tubes with my patient's blood.

"I just wanted to stop by and check on things. I came in with the guy next door—the gunshot to the chest—and saw you in here. We'll do what we can about getting some officers over here. But it's gonna be awhile."

He spun around and was gone. And I was nervous. There had been fights in the waiting room following high-school football games and minor rumbles in town. But this was something worse—something bigger than any of that.

"I'm here if you need anything, Doc."

I looked at the doorway and there stood Willis Barber, our nighttime security guard. Willis was a great guy, but he was at least seventy, skinny as a November stalk of corn, and unarmed.

Now I was *really* nervous, but I was able to force a nod and a smile.

"Seems to be getting a little out of hand in the waiting room." He shifted his weight from one foot to the other and stroked his gray, stubbled chin. "I'll go see what I can do."

Willis stepped into the hallway, turned to his left—the opposite direction from the waiting room—and disappeared. We didn't see him the rest of the night.

The OR crew came for my patient and wheeled him out of the department. I had just reached the nurses' station when the ambulance-entrance doors blew open and EMS 3 brought two stretchers into the ER.

"This one's cut up pretty bad," one of the paramedics gasped, breathing hard. "And the other has a stab wound of his belly. He thinks butcher knife."

"Take the stab wound into major," Virginia commanded from the triage entrance. "And the lacerations back to minor trauma."

The paramedic nodded without a word and the stretchers sped smoothly past us.

Virginia stepped over to my side. "It's pretty tense in the waiting room. I've moved as many of our regular patients and their families as I could to the back hallway, but we're running out of space. No police officers, and the fight looks like it's spreading this way. There's something going on in the parking lot, right outside the entrance. A lot of yelling and pushing. I've got a three-year-old with fever and an earache that I need to get back. He's scared to death."

She paused, adjusted her bifocals, and chuckled. "Have to admit, I'm a little worried myself. This powder keg could explode any minute."

Twenty minutes later, it *did* explode. Whatever had been going on in the parking lot spilled through the ER entrance and into the waiting room. Four young men were swinging at each other—fortunately no guns were involved—and chairs were flying. They weren't doing much damage to each other, and the altercation quickly flowed back through the entrance and out into the parking lot again.

"Anything I can do, Dr. Lesslie?"

I turned around and was face-to-face with Ansel Pardee. Ansel worked with the hospital's housekeeping department and was a kind, generous, soft-spoken man—a friend to everyone. Part of his assignment tonight was the ER. Amy must have called him for major trauma. It was still a mess.

"Thanks, Ansel. Maybe in major."

Ansel was a little taller than me—probably six-two—and solid as a rock. He was leaning on a broom and smiling at me. *What had he told me about retiring? He was almost sixty-five and getting close.*

"Dr. Lesslie, we've got a problem."

What now?

Behind me stood Alberta Fleming, one of our overnight registration secretaries. She worked out front, separated from the waiting area by a low, narrow desk.

Her eyes were open wide and she was trembling.

"About twenty men—maybe twenty-five—just came in, demanding to see their cousin. I think they're talking about the young man with the gunshot wound of his abdomen. I've asked them to have a seat or wait outside, but they're just standing there milling around. It's getting ugly. They won't leave, and say they'll just find a way to get back here." She stopped, leaned close to me, and whispered. "And Dr. Lesslie, I'm pretty sure a couple of them have guns."

I spun around to Amy. She was standing behind the counter, phone pressed to her ear and her hand covering the mouthpiece. "I've got Sergeant Bridgers on the line but he can't get anyone over here for twenty or thirty minutes."

"Let me step out there." Ansel Pardee's voice was calm, measured. Before I could say anything he disappeared through the triage door.

I turned back to Amy. She still had the phone pressed to her ear. She shook her head and didn't say a word.

"Heaven help us." Alberta spun around and scurried back to her front desk.

"Dr. Lesslie, I need you in here, right now." Virginia disappeared back into major. I recognized the tone of her voice and bolted after her.

Fifteen minutes later, our butcher-knife patient was stabilized and I walked over to the nurses' station.

"Amy, can you get the OR on the phone? We need to let them know what's next."

I grabbed a piece of paper, scribbled a few notes, and froze.

Ansel Pardee! What had I been thinking? He was out in the waiting room all alone.

I hurried through triage and opened the waiting-room door. There was Ansel, standing in the middle of the room with his broom, sweeping some loose pieces of trash. Two or three people sat quietly in chairs, watching the wall-mounted TV.

He looked up and gave me a big grin.

"Ansel, what did…how did you…?"

He chuckled and motioned me over to his side. Leaning close, he whispered, "Doc, I came out here, saw all those hooligans, and picked out the one I thought was the ringleader. I walked up to him and got right in his face. Just stood there for a while, starin' at him. Then I said, 'Son, I know your momma.' And that was that."

Ansel winked at me, grabbed his broom, and started sweeping again.

I heard him whistling as I walked back through the triage door.

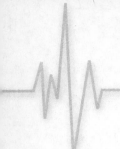

On Silent Wings They Come

"What do you think? We're only two minutes away."

Paramedics Mike and Sharon Brothers were in the ambulance of EMS 3, returning to Rock Hill on Highway 161. Their police scanner had buzzed to life—the dispatcher calling for any available unit to respond to a forced breaking and entering.

"She didn't mention any personal injuries," Sharon answered her husband. "They probably don't need us. If they do, they'll call."

"Yeah, but we're close. Let's check it out."

A few minutes later, the ambulance turned off 161 and onto a well-kept graveled road. A final curve, and there was the house—well-guarded by clumps of pine trees and cedars. A county sheriff's patrol car was parked on some patchy grass, its blue lights still flashing.

A loud blast from behind the stopped ambulance startled Sharon.

"What in the world! I think I wet my pants!"

She jumped out the passenger door and waved a fist at the approaching fire engine. Andy West was driving and he laughed, shaking his head and pointing at the paramedic.

He blew his horn once more, just for good measure, and brought the unit to a stop.

Deputy Lou Warner walked over to the ambulance and stood beside Mike.

"These poor folks. This is the worst I've ever seen." He pointed toward the house and to a man and woman who stood near the front door, talking with another officer. A little girl, probably four years old, stood by her mother's side and clutched one of the woman's legs with both arms.

"What happened?" Sharon stepped over to the two men, glancing over her shoulder at the parked fire engine, lest Andy let loose another blast.

Lou shook his head and jammed his hands into his coat pockets. It was a week after Thanksgiving and the temperature was close to freezing. "Somebody broke into the house while they weren't at home. The whole family was across town at the Walmart and was only gone for a couple of hours. When they got back, this is what they found. Come on, I'll show you."

Mike and Lou headed toward the newly constructed vinyl-sided house. Sharon hesitated. She was only a hundred feet away and just now noticed the front door.

Odd. It's freezing out here, but the door is wide open. Wait—

The door wasn't just open—it had been ripped from its hinges and stood leaning against its splintered wooden frame.

Mike looked over his shoulder. "Come on, Sharon."

She quickly caught up to the two men and stepped onto the small cement stoop. Lou's partner was a few yards to her right, still talking to the couple and their daughter, making notes on a small flip pad.

Sharon wiped her feet on a rubber doormat. Its Christmas greeting— NOEL—was almost completely obscured by the red mud of the sparsely grassed front yard. She was about to follow Lou and Mike into the house when she noticed the little boy standing under a window twenty feet from the stoop.

He was by himself, bundled against the cold December air, with his bright-red stocking cap pulled low over his ears. His mittened hands hung limply by his side and he was staring at something on the ground.

It was a pumpkin—smashed into sad, pulpy pieces. In spite of the biting cold, Sharon's face flushed a bright red.

"Are you coming?" Mike called out again.

The small living room was completely destroyed. The remains of a few wooden chairs were scattered on the floor and the one lonely piece of furniture—a dark brown and worn Naugahyde lounge chair—had been turned on its side and repeatedly slashed.

"Whoever did this meant business." Lou was pointing to a far wall, next to the kitchen. The Sheetrock had been ripped off and was scattered in dusty pieces on the floor. "They knew what they were doing. This is a new house, and they were hoping to find copper pipes. Same thing in the bathrooms. The whole place is a wreck."

"Why the chair?" Sharon glanced at the floor behind her. "Why would someone cut it up like that?"

"Just plain meanness," Lou answered.

"I'm just glad nobody was home." Mike shook his head and stepped into the small kitchen.

"Yeah, somebody might have gotten hurt." Lou glanced through the open front door at the small family.

"Looks like they took everything in this room." Mike kicked away some debris from where the refrigerator had once stood. Any appliances—anything of value was gone. "How did they do this in only a couple of hours?"

"We've seen it happen before," Lou answered. "They drive up in a truck and start ripping stuff out and loading it up. They don't waste any time."

Sharon thought about the smashed pumpkin. Someone had taken the time to make *that* statement.

Gary and Kimberly Fields had finished talking with Lou's partner. He motioned to Deputy Warner and they headed for the patrol car.

"See you guys later," Lou said to Mike and Sharon.

He stopped beside the couple and their little girl. "I'm really sorry about this. We're going to do everything we can to find the people who did it."

Gary Fields nodded slowly, glanced at his ruined home, and quickly looked away.

"Thank you, Officer." Kimberly managed a pained smile and called to her son. "Mark, come here. You and Hannah need to start cleaning up your rooms."

She took a few steps toward the gaping front entrance, and had to stop. Fireman Andy West was standing in the doorway, completely blocking it.

"Ma'am, I'm afraid you're not going to be able to stay here."

Kimberly's mouth dropped and her face flamed to a fire-engine red.

"But…this is our home! Where are we supposed to go? This is the only…"

"Ma'am, I'm sorry." Andy spoke quietly, and looked down at his heavy boots. "We don't have a choice. It's dangerous, and there's no power—no water. You just can't stay here."

Kimberly turned to her husband, question marks firing from her eyes. He hung his head.

A few days later, Mike and Sharon were starting an early breakfast at Anna J's, having just finished their twenty-four-hour shift.

"More coffee?" their waitress asked.

"I'll have some," Lou Warner said from behind the young woman, startling her. "And Mike, you can slide over. I'm hungry."

The deputy sheriff sat down and ordered breakfast. He handed the menu to the waitress and settled back into the comfortable booth.

Sharon stirred butter into her grits. "Any word on those folks who had their house broken into?"

"The Fields family? We've got a couple of leads, but nothing solid yet. We'll find 'em."

Lou sat up straight, folded his arms on the table, and shook his head.

"That was their dream house, you know. They moved up here a couple of years ago from some small town in Georgia. Gary—the father—was working two jobs, trying to save up enough money for a down payment. His wife wanted to get a job too. But he insisted on her staying home with the kids. Hannah, the girl, is four and Mark is five, I think. Anyway, they saved up enough to buy a little piece of property and get started on a small house. I think one of the local contractors helped them out. They had only been in the place a couple of months."

The waitress stepped to the table with a steaming plate and Lou leaned back, giving her room to set it down.

"Where are they staying now?" Sharon asked.

Lou surveyed his breakfast—a fork in one hand and his coffee mug in the other.

"No family anywhere near," he answered. "But they've managed to find a room at one of the motels on Riverview Road. To make matters worse, that old truck of theirs broke down as soon as they got to the motel and they can't afford to get it fixed. It's a half hour away. Gary can walk to his first job, but he has to catch a ride every day to his second one. They're stranded—stuck."

"What about the house?" Mike wiped his mouth with a napkin and dropped it onto his empty plate.

"No insurance, no money. It's just sitting there with the doors boarded up. The whole thing is really sad." Lou paused and sighed heavily. "But what are you going to do?"

"I'll tell you what we're going to do." Sharon slid to the end of the booth, stood up, and looked down at her husband. "Come on, Mike. I've got an idea."

Sharon and Mike Brothers, together with Lou Warner, Andy West, and a bunch of their friends, decided on a plan. Some in the group had carpentry skills, some were part-time electricians and plumbers, and Sharon could cook. For the next three weekends, these big-hearted and selfless volunteers would descend upon the desolate house on that lonely graveled road. Soon, it was transformed once again into a warm, inviting home.

"No reason they can't stay here now." Andy West smiled at the group and taped a "certificate of occupancy" to the brand-new front door. A control box was fastened to a wall just inside and he tapped it a few times. "And now they have an alarm system—hooked up direct to the County."

They were admiring their handiwork when the blaring, obnoxious horn of an approaching vehicle caused them to turn and stare. An old Dodge van cleared the last of the cedar trees, drove toward the house, and came to a sudden stop right in front of them.

Sharon Brothers jumped from the driver's side—key in hand, arms waving.

"Look what we have!"

A member of her church heard what was going on and had donated one of his used vehicles.

"Ted Wiley sends his regards!" she told the group. "He even threw in two extra tires and twenty dollars for gas."

"Let's go get the Fields!" someone shouted. "We're ready, aren't we?"

Sharon and Lou were elected to drive into town and pick up the Fields family. They knocked on the motel room door, let Gary and Kimberly know they had a surprise for them, and told them to pack up some clothes—and to not ask any questions.

Gravel complained and crunched under the van's tires as the Dodge slowly approached the house. Gary and Kimberly stared with wide eyes and open mouths at their front yard.

"Mama, who are all those people?" Mark, their little boy, had rolled down his window and was leaning out of the van.

Twenty waving and hollering people stood in front of the Fields' home.

"Merry Christmas!"

Mark and Hannah jumped out and ran toward the cheering group. Gary and Kimberly slowly got out of the van, put their arms around each other, and took a few hesitant steps.

They stopped, tears flowing down their cheeks, and could only shake their heads.

There were only a few days remaining before Christmas. Mike and Sharon were sitting at their kitchen table, drinking coffee.

"Did you see any toys or Christmas presents when we moved the Fields into their house?" Sharon asked her husband.

Mike leaned back in his chair and shook his head. "Don't remember any. Why?"

"Come on—let's go." Sharon jumped up and headed toward the backdoor.

Her hand was on the doorknob but Mike was still sitting, staring at his wife.

"I said, come on."

After a trip to Walmart and Target, they were headed toward the Fields' house.

"Just how are we going to do this?" Mike asked. "You said you wanted to surprise them."

"Don't you worry. I've got a plan."

They drove out to the Fields' home and just after turning onto the graveled road, Sharon shut off the engine.

"This is close enough. Let's get the stuff."

Mike shook his head and followed orders.

Dozens of merrily wrapped packages sprawled in the back of their SUV. It was all they could do to secure them in their arms and still be able to see where they were going.

They slowly made their way toward the house, occasionally scrambling to keep some of the gifts from falling to the ground. Finally, they cleared the last group of cedars. A lighted Christmas tree could be seen through the living-room window, but there was no movement—no sign of anyone who would detect their presence.

"Come on," Sharon whispered. "Let's go."

They veered toward the left side of the house, then edged along the front to the small stoop.

"Put 'em down here, but be quiet." Sharon began stacking her packages, building a whimsical, brightly colored pyramid.

Mike carefully placed the last small box on the top of the pile. "That's it. Let's get going before someone comes out."

They retraced their furtive steps, got fifty feet from the house, and took off running.

Sharon started giggling and Mike shushed her.

Neither of them saw the brown-eyed, towheaded boy peeping at them from a front bedroom window.

It was a week after Christmas, and Hannah Fields was sick. Her parents brought her to the ER and Lori Davidson took her back to the ENT room. The note on the chart was typical for the season:

Fever, crying, earache.

Thankfully, it was something simple—a routine ear infection—and I told Kimberly and Gary what we needed to do.

"Did you guys have a good Christmas?" I asked, looking at the two children. I didn't know anything about the "special delivery."

Hannah had sat with her head hanging and lower lip sticking out the entire time. When she heard me say "Christmas" everything changed. She started smiling and bouncing on the stretcher.

"Santa came to our house! Santa came!"

Gary looked at his wife and raised his eyebrows.

"It was the best Christmas *ever!*" Mark chimed in. "*Ever!*"

"That's great." I tousled his light brown hair and looked up at his parents. "I'll write those prescriptions and one of the nurses will be right back."

One of the EMS units had brought in a possible hip fracture and I was talking to the two paramedics at the nurses' station.

Lori had taken Hannah's prescriptions to ENT and I heard her coming up the hall with the Fields family.

I turned in their direction and watched as she led the parade toward us. Hannah was being carried by her father, and Mark was hanging back a little, playing with one of his Christmas games. The boy stopped, energetically pushed a couple of buttons, then shook his head and sighed.

He looked up, took a few hurried steps trying to catch up with his parents, and suddenly froze in the middle of the hallway. His eyes widened and he pointed in my direction.

"Mama! Daddy! It's Santa Claus!"

I glanced behind me. Mark was pointing to Mike Brothers—and his blushing helper.

A Time to Be Born…

It was almost dusk, and the light was quickly fading. Its scattered beams penetrated the deep woods at the back of the ER parking lot and settled comfortably on a dogwood tree growing in a natural area near the ambulance entrance. *The* dogwood tree.

Camille Anderson was forty-two years old. You would never guess it if you got a close look at her. I wouldn't. I thought she was in her mid to late twenties—thirty at the most. Her face and skin were radiant, set off by bright, sparkling eyes. And that constant smile, always outlined by bright-red, flawlessly applied lipstick.

"She looks like an angel," one of her patients once remarked.

She might have been. One thing for sure, she was a great ER nurse—caring, observant, always helpful, and patient. Well, *usually* patient. She would occasionally let you know of her displeasure if she felt someone was being mistreated, especially if that someone was a child or an older person.

The angriest I had ever seen her was on a Sunday afternoon. This is almost always a busy time in the ER. After church, family members would visit their loved ones residing in "retirement" homes, find them in some worrisome state, and have them brought to the emergency department for an evaluation. Their primary-care doctors weren't available and it fell to us to try to sort things out. Usually it was something simple and straightforward. Occasionally it was something worse.

On this particular Sunday afternoon, it was something worse. An elderly gentleman had been brought in by his children because of what they thought were some infected insect bites on his arms and legs. The staff of the nursing home had tried to cover these up with hastily applied bandages, but weren't successful. The man's son had seen the wounds and became suspicious when he received evasive answers from the staff. He put his father in the car and brought him to us to be examined.

"These are starting to get infected." I leaned close and gently touched the skin surrounding these scattered pencil-eraser-sized marks. The elderly man didn't say anything, but pulled his injured arm away from me. There were dozens of these wounds on his other arm and on his legs.

Camille was standing beside me. Her eyes were open wide and her bright-red lips were trembling. She knew.

"These look like cigarette burns," I told the son. "And they need to be taken care of. I don't think he should be going back to that retirement home."

His son's face turned a chalky white and his mouth fell open. "Cigarette burns? You mean someone has—"

Camille spun around and bolted out of the room. I knew where she was headed, and I also knew there were no retirement home staff members here for her to confront. They were fortunate.

A few minutes later, I walked over to the nurses' station and overheard Camille's telephone conversation.

"That's right, Officer. This is the ER and we need someone over here right now to investigate an assault—abuse—whatever. Just get over here!"

She slammed the phone down, turned around, and looked at me. Her face was flushed and I could see the struggle in her eyes. She took a deep breath, flattened the front of her dress with the palms of her hands, stood up straight, and said, "Okay, I need to go take care of that gentleman's burns."

That was the rare exception, but when she was on fire, we all knew to stand back and just let it happen. At all other times, Camille was a bright spot in what could be a stressful and trying environment. Her spirit was calming, and I frequently sought her out to help calm my own.

Such was the case one Tuesday morning. We hadn't been that busy, but every patient who came in was very involved and complicated. I was getting frazzled and noticed Camille stepping into the medicine room. I followed, and walked up behind her as she was drawing up some medicine for one of our patients.

She looked up at me and shook her head. "Take a deep breath, Dr. Lesslie. We're going to make it." Camille cocked her head and gave me a two-fingered salute—her trademark.

She smiled and turned back to her work. That was all I had needed—just a moment with Camille and the quiet retreat of the medicine room.

I looked over her shoulder and out into the parking lot. Twenty or thirty yards from the window was a small natural area, in the middle of which stood a dogwood tree. It was January, and its leaves had long since fallen, leaving it bare and forlorn.

"See that tree out there? The dogwood?"

Camille looked up and leaned closer to the window. "Yes, the one over in the pine needles?" She was pointing to the natural area.

"That's it. Now I want you to take a good look at that tree. See how bare it is? How lonely?"

"It's bare alright, Dr. Lesslie. It's the middle of winter. What's gotten into you?" She turned around, still smiling, but her eyes squinted and she tilted her head.

"Here's what we're going to do." I was feeling philosophical and didn't miss a beat. "This April or May, you and I are going to meet in this room and look at that tree again. It will be blossoming and putting on new leaves—totally different from the way it looks now."

"I get it." Her face relaxed and her eyes twinkled. "Like the circle of life—changes of season—that kind of stuff."

"Right. That kind of stuff. Let's see if we can remember to do that."

"Hmm, hmm. Okay, let's just see." She picked up the medication syringe and walked out of the room.

We did remember, or at least Camille did. It was the end of April, and early one morning she motioned for me to come over to the medication room. She was standing near the window, hands on hips, and grinning. She nodded and I looked over her shoulder, out into the parking area.

There it was, in full glory. The dogwood tree was covered in white, cross-shaped blossoms, and its young, just-visible leaves promised a green and glorious spring.

"You were right, Dr. Lesslie. It's come alive—been reborn. Isn't it beautiful?"

We stood beside each other and silently looked at the dogwood. We were in the midst of a busy, bustling ER, but here was our reality. Here was a rare moment of peace.

The next time I looked at the dogwood tree, really contemplated it, was the following December. Its limbs were once again bare, desolate.

I stood alone in the medicine room, lost in my thoughts. Camille wouldn't be joining me to mark the passing of another season, another dying to be followed by rebirth. Two weeks earlier, she had collapsed in her front yard, dead from a massive stroke. Camille, gone. How could that be?

The lifeless branches of the dogwood swayed erratically in the cold winter wind.

─────ᨓᨓ─────

It was Amy Connors who pointed it out.

"You know who that is, don't you?" She nodded toward a young woman walking out through the ambulance entrance. Tightly clutching her right hand was the three-year-old little girl I had just treated for an ear infection.

The doors closed behind them and I turned to Amy. "No, who are they?"

"That's Camille Anderson's daughter and granddaughter. I thought you knew."

I *didn't* know, and I dropped the chart in my hand and hurried out into the parking lot, trying to catch up with them.

"Ma'am." I called after them, not remembering the mother's name.

She stopped and turned around, the little girl staring up at me with large, dark eyes and a huge smile.

"Yes, did we forget something?"

"No, I just wanted to tell you—your mother, Camille, was a special lady. We're all sorry about what happened, and we really miss her."

She sighed and her chin dropped to her chest. But only for a moment. She looked up at me with a smile—one I had seen before on her mother's face—and said, "She loved working in the ER, and she loved the staff here. And...we miss her too."

She looked down at her daughter and sighed again. "Thanks."

The little girl grinned, cocked her head, and gave me a two-fingered salute.

They turned and walked out into the parking lot. I watched for a moment, glad for the chance to talk with her, and headed back to the ER.

I stopped just outside the entrance and looked to my right.

The dogwood tree. It was covered in white blossoms and young green leaves.

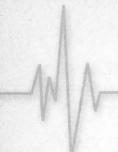

Pokie

An October Friday night—10:47 p.m. "Isn't that Coach Jeffers?" Amy Connors nodded toward the back of the department, and I twisted around.

"Yeah, it is." No one living in Rock Hill could miss the towering, muscular frame of one of the state's leading football coaches, even with his back to us. He disappeared into the ortho room and I turned back to Amy. "What's he doing here?"

"Jackson Alexander is here with an injured wrist." Jeff Ryan walked over to the nurses' station and put three empty clipboards on the countertop. "Took him back to ortho while you were in cardiac with the heart attack."

"That's right." I suddenly remembered it was Friday night, and Coach Jeffers's team had its first playoff game. Jackson Alexander was the star quarterback. Though only a sophomore, he was already being heavily recruited for college.

I glanced at the clock on the wall. The game should be over by now.

"How did it turn out?" I asked Jeff.

"Well, we won, but it was close. And mighty scary." He leaned against the counter and propped an elbow on the laminate surface. "Jackson went down early in the fourth quarter with a hurt wrist and couldn't go back in. He's in X-ray now. If it's broken, the chances of winning any more games are almost zero. That's why Coach Jeffers is here, I'm sure. He's checkin' on him."

Twenty minutes later, I was standing in front of the X-ray view box, studying the films of Jackson Alexander's right wrist—his throwing hand.

Breathing down my neck—actually down on the top of my head— was Coach Jeffers. He was flanked by Jackson on one side and the boy's parents on the other.

"What do you think, Doc? Everything okay?" The coach leaned close and put a huge hand on my shoulder.

I looked the X-rays over for the fifth time. Nothing. There was no fracture.

A loud *whoop* followed my announcement, and then a probable A-C separation when the coach pounded my shoulder.

We put Jackson's wrist in a splint for a couple of days and sent the elated group home. He would be fine by next Friday night, ready to play.

"Now that's one happy bunch of folks." Amy leaned back in her chair and slapped her hands on the desk.

Jeff Ryan walked around the nurses' station and sat down heavily in the chair beside Amy. "There'll be a *bunch* of happy folks in Rock Hill when they find out he's okay."

I rubbed my shoulder and said, "I'm just glad nothing was *broken*."

"Yep," Amy grinned. "That was pure joy on their faces when they heard the news."

Virginia Granger walked out of the medicine room and over to our small group.

"What exactly do you mean by 'pure joy,' Amy?" The heard nurse pulled a chair from under the desk, sat down, and studied her secretary.

"You know…They were…happy—real glad that he wasn't hurt. Pure joy."

Virginia removed her bifocals, took a small handkerchief from her dress pocket, and carefully cleaned them.

"Happy, for sure," she said quietly. "Relieved too. But I'm not sure about the 'joy' part. I think that would be something different."

I watched Virginia closely as she slowly fitted her glasses on her nose and looked over at Amy. *Where was she going with this?*

"What's the difference?" Amy hunched her shoulders and glanced at me. "Happy—glad—joyful. Aren't they all the same?"

"There's a difference, I think," Virginia began. "Joy—true joy—is something special. Something rare. Lots of things can make us happy and glad. Many times, those things are superficial and not really impor-tant. Those emotions quickly pass. But joy, that's something from way· down deep, from somewhere in our hearts."

She stopped and looked beyond us, down the hallway.

"*There's* someone who knows the difference."

We all turned and looked to the back of the department. Ansel Pardee, a sixty-four-year-old member of the hospital's housekeeping department, was walking toward us, mop in one hand and bucket in the other. His eyes met ours and a huge grin spread across his face. *When had I not seen this man without a huge grin?*

Ansel gave us a nod and disappeared into minor trauma.

"Ansel's a great guy," Amy said, shifting in her seat and turning toward Virginia. "He's always happy and ready to help—ready to do anything he can for us. I've never seen him upset about anything—always smilin'. But what do you mean? Why isn't *that* having joy? What's the difference?"

Virginia settled back in her chair. "You've seen his grandson before, haven't you?"

"Yeah, sure." Amy nodded. "Little Pokie."

"That's right—Little Pokie."

~~~

Ansel Pardee had just buried his wife when their daughter, Jasmine, gave birth to his first and only grandchild. The boy was named after his father, Malcolm, but he was in prison when the child was born, and Ansel couldn't—or wouldn't—bring himself to use that name. He had never approved of his daughter seeing Malcolm, but she was headstrong and hadn't been willing to listen to his concerns or her mother's.

"Jasmine was a difficult child," Virginia said in understatement. "Dropped out of high school when she was seventeen and started hanging out with the wrong crowd. That's how she met Malcolm. Then she was pregnant, and her mother got sick. When she died, Jasmine went off the deep end. That was a difficult time for Ansel, as you can imagine. But you'd never know it. He had the same smile and peaceful nature then as he does now."

She paused and shook her head. "It was Dr. Alexis, their pediatrician, who discovered the boy had HIV. I remember talking with Ansel right after he found out. He was worried, but told me the Lord would help his grandchild, and he would find some way to get him the best medical help possible. It was like a light went on with Ansel. He bonded with that child in a way that…in a way I've never seen. That's about the time he gave him his new name—Pokie."

"How did he ever come up with '*Pokie*'?" Amy chuckled.

"Well, the little chap was quite precocious and was walking way before he was one year old. He was unsteady, of course, and a little slow. Ansel would hold out his arms and say, 'Come on, Pokie,' and the name stuck. He's been 'Pokie' ever since."

Virginia's smile disappeared and she shook her head. "When that light came on for Ansel—that special bond between him and Pokie—it went out for Jasmine. Something in her mind just flipped, and her drug and alcohol problems got worse. She had a couple of close brushes with the law and then she was gone. Ansel hasn't heard from her in more than four years. He's not even sure she's still alive. He's been raising the boy as if he were his own son."

We were silent for a moment, then Jeff asked, "What about Malcolm, the kid's father?"

Virginia took a deep breath and sighed. "There's the rub. He got out of prison six or seven months ago and came back to Rock Hill. He told Ansel he was a changed man and wanted to raise his son. You can imagine what Ansel thought, but there was nothing he could do. The courts were on Malcolm's side, and he and Pokie moved in with Malcolm's mother. Ansel would visit when he could, but Malcolm made it difficult."

"Wait a minute!" Amy sat bolt upright in her chair. "Six or seven months ago...It was about four months ago that Pokie came to the ER with a broken collarbone. Remember? The story was he had fallen down a couple of steps."

"That's right." Virginia nodded slowly. "That was the *first* time. And then there was the laceration on the top of his head. I can't remember the reason Malcolm gave for that injury."

"The *excuse*, you mean," Jeff interjected. "I was here the night Malcolm's mother brought Pokie in with a broken arm. We called the police and DSS. *You* called the police, as I remember it." He looked at Virginia. "You were the first to know what was going on."

"No, not me." She shook her head and looked down the hall. "It was Ansel. Malcolm's mother had called him and said they were on the way to the ER. He got here before they did. *He* knew what was happening, and he told me he was going to put a stop to it once and for all. That's why I called the police. Ansel is a peaceful man, but you know how big he is—and strong as an ox. When it came to his Pokie, anything could happen."

"I was standing right here." Jeff turned and looked at the ambulance entrance. "Right in this spot, when Malcolm stomped through those doors. It was a perfect storm. Pokie, his grandmother, and Ansel had just gotten back from X-ray and were standing right over there with a police officer." He paused and pointed to the wall beside the cardiac room. "The woman from DSS was standing right beside them, writing up her report. Malcolm was drunk and hollerin' and demanded that Ansel hand over his son. When he reached out for the boy, the police officer—smoothest thing I've ever seen—slapped his handcuffs on Malcolm, spun him around, and marched him out the door. Just like that, and he was gone."

"Not been back, either," Virginia added. "They had been investigating the case and had already decided to give Ansel custody of Pokie. That incident only cemented the deal. The woman from DSS told Ansel that night, and said he could take Pokie home with him—that Malcolm had no further claim to the boy. I've never seen a man hug a child so— Well, nobody was going to take him out of his arms."

She leaned back in her chair and smiled at Amy.

"I understand now," Amy said quietly. "The look on Ansel's face that night—*that* was pure joy."

Virginia nodded. "It *was*, Amy—it was pure joy. But that wasn't all."

Her voice broke and she looked away. When she turned around, there were tears in her eyes.

"It was also the look on Pokie's face."

THE *Miracle* OF
FORGIVENESS

We are most like beasts when we kill.
We are most like men when we judge.
We are most like God when we forgive.

WILLIAM ARTHUR WARD (1921–1994)

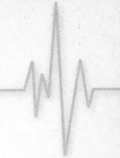

It's Okay

Virginia Granger walked up behind Charlotte and put a hand on the younger woman's shoulder. "I've got this one. See if you can help Dr. Stevens back in ortho. I think he has a fractured wrist to take care of."

Charlotte Turner looked at her head nurse, and then her eyes started darting around the department, finally coming to rest on the closed ambulance entrance doors.

EMS 2 was on the way in with a seventeen-year-old male, the victim of an auto accident out on Highway 21. It didn't sound very good—head injury, crushed chest. "ETOH on board," the paramedic reported. The teenager had been drinking.

Charlotte was assigned major trauma and would normally be taking care of this patient when he arrived. Virginia had something else in mind. Charlotte was a good ER nurse, but she wasn't ready for this. Not yet.

"It's alright, Mrs. Granger. I'll—"

"I want you back in ortho." There was no mistaking the intent of her words, or her gently taking the younger nurse by the shoulders and directing her down the hallway. "We'll be fine here. I think I remember how to help Dr. Lesslie."

I was standing in the doorway, watching all of this and waiting for EMS 2.

"Thanks, Virginia," I said quietly. "That was going to be tough."

Charlotte walked slowly down the hall, glancing briefly over her shoulder at the ambulance doors. This was still hard for her—and had been since that night six months earlier.

It was midnight on an October Friday, and the "A Team" was on duty. Lori Davidson, Charlotte Turner, and Jeff Ryan were the nurses, and Amy

Connors was sitting behind the nurses' station, making sure everything ran smoothly. My job was to stay out of their way.

"ER, this is EMS 1." Denton Roberts's voice shattered the hard-fought-for calm of the department.

"EMS 1, this is the ER. Go ahead." Lori had the receiver in one hand, pen in the other, ready to make some notes on the pad in front of her.

"Five minutes out with a one-car 10-50. Is...Dr. Lesslie nearby?"

My head jerked in the direction of the radio. A 10-50—auto accident. *Why would Denton need to talk with me?*

"He's standing right here, EMS 1. Go ahead." Lori looked over at me and shrugged.

"Can you give him the radio and switch off the speakerphone?"

"What in the world?" Amy said quietly, looking at Lori and then over to me.

"Must be something bad." Charlotte had just walked over from triage and was leaning against the counter.

I nodded, and Lori said, "Okay, EMS 1, here's Dr. Lesslie."

She flipped the speakerphone switch and handed me the receiver. Amy leaned close to me, straining her neck to hear.

Something was up, and I stepped away from the desk and turned my back.

"Denton, this is Dr. Lesslie. Go ahead."

"Doc, I saw Charlotte Turner in the ER earlier tonight. Is she still there?"

Denton's voice was quiet, hesitant. Something was troubling him. I turned around and looked at Charlotte and my heart jumped into my throat. I looked away before she could see the blood draining from my face. I knew.

"Yes, still here. What's going on?"

"This 10-50, it's—the driver is a seventeen-year-old kid, and he's fine. Drunk, but fine. The passenger—he wasn't belted and was ejected from the car. Head and chest injuries and what looks like a broken neck." Denton paused, and the silence was stifling. "Doc, it's Charlotte's boy, Russell. And he's dead."

I looked up again at Charlotte and our eyes met. She was talking with Lori, and smiling about something Amy had just said. She froze, staring at me.

"What is it, Dr. Lesslie? What's the matter?"

Amy spun around and looked at me. Then she looked at Charlotte and down at the radio.

"Oh Lord."

Denton never brought Russell's body into the department. He called the coroner and took him straight to the morgue where Charlotte, her husband, and I were now headed. They would have to identify the body of their son. Lori was already there with Denton and the coroner.

They struggled forward as we walked down the quiet, lonely hallways in the back of the hospital. And then we were there, standing just outside the closed doors of the hospital morgue. Charlotte's knees buckled, and her husband grabbed her just before she collapsed into the wall. They looked at each other, pushed the door open, and walked inside.

We slowly made our way back to the ER. Charlotte and her husband had their arms around each other and shuffled along as if on some powerful hypnotic drug. As we passed the doorway of minor trauma, they both looked in and suddenly stopped. Sitting on the back left stretcher, his head hanging and his feet dangling, was Bobby Green, their son's friend and the driver of the demolished car.

Bobby looked up and into the eyes of the Turners. Charlotte shrank against her husband, and he took a step toward the door, his shoulders suddenly tense.

I stepped between them and the cowering teenager in minor. "Let's go to the nurses' station. We need to talk about a couple of things."

Reluctantly, Charlotte's husband gave ground, and we headed again up the hallway. Jeff Ryan met us at the desk. I leaned over and whispered, "Make sure the kid stays in minor." He nodded, and quickly headed in that direction.

The ambulance doors opened. It was Virginia Granger, and she headed straight for Charlotte. She took the nurse in her arms and the two women held each other tightly, rocking from side to side. Lori and I looked away.

———

And now, six months later, we were once again dealing with teenage tragedy. Virginia and I took care of the young man in major trauma, and Charlotte stayed back in ortho with Dr. Stephens until long after the patient had been transferred to another hospital.

She seemed okay, but the sadness in her eyes remained. We waited and hoped for the sparkle to return and for her to find some measure of peace. It was over a year in coming, but it finally happened.

~~~

I was in minor stitching the finger of a teenage boy, making small talk as the final suture was being knotted. He had been sharpening a lawn mower and the blade had slipped—and here he was. We talked about sports, about his plans after graduating that spring, about where catgut thread came from. I didn't put two and two together.

Charlotte Turner had walked into minor and was standing behind me, looking over my shoulder at the young man on the stretcher. I had asked him a question but he didn't answer. Intent on what I was doing, I didn't look up, and repeated myself.

When he still didn't respond, I rolled back on the stool and looked up at him. He was staring behind me with eyes wide, the blood draining from his face.

I twisted around to face Charlotte, and then looked back at my patient.

What in the—My eyes shot to the chart lying on the stretcher beside him.

Bobby Green.

I should have noticed. This was the young man who was driving the night Charlotte's son, Russell, was killed. I kept tying knots in that last stitch, desperately trying to think of what was the best thing for me to do.

"Mrs. Turner..." Bobby was struggling, his voice quiet and breaking. "I want you to know that—"

Charlotte stepped around me and over to the side of the stretcher. She looked down at Bobby and their eyes met. They stayed like that, motionless, until finally she reached out and put a hand on his shoulder.

"It's okay." Her voice was soft, gentle. "It's okay, Bobby."

His head slumped to his chest and he reached up and put his hand on hers. And then it began. His body shook with deep, painful sobs.

It was done. With those few, simple words she had released him.

And by doing so, she had released herself.

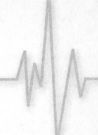

Forgive Us Our Trespasses...

"Is the coroner here yet?"

Amy Connors looked up at me from behind the nurses' station and shook her head. "He's on the way. Maybe another fifteen or twenty minutes."

I turned and glanced at the closed door of major trauma. Lori Davidson was still in there with the Grissoms—and their dead son.

Officer Jody Bridges and his partner had been the first to arrive at the scene. It was a little after midnight, and pouring down rain. Visibility was terrible, and they had almost missed the twisted pile of metal wrapped around a large oak tree, barely twenty feet off the road.

Eighteen-year-old Reed Levin had been easy to find. He was trapped in the driver's seat by the distended airbag. He was moaning, moving his arms, and seemed to be stable and largely uninjured– except for the blood that streamed from an obviously broken nose.

When Reed saw Jody's bouncing flashlight beam approaching the wrecked car, he began calling out for Case. Over and over. "Case!"

His partner checked on Reed, trying to calm him down, while Jody played his light over the empty front passenger seat and the mangled passenger door—twisted on its hinges and sprawling open.

"This kid's not wearing a seat belt," his partner said. "Lucky that his airbag deployed. Looks like it kept him from being thrown out."

Jody's light searched for the passenger belt. It was unlatched and stuffed into the sides of the seat.

The blaring siren of EMS 1 seemed muffled by the rain as the ambulance turned a curve in the road. The two paramedics caught sight of the blue flashing lights of the patrol car, slowed their speeding vehicle, and pulled off the road just to its side. They bolted from the ambulance, leaving the motor running and their lights flooding the eerie, rain-drenched scene.

"What have you got?" Denton Roberts, the lead paramedic, asked Jody.

The officer told him what they had found.

"Case!" Reed's cry pierced the pitch-black darkness. "Case!"

"There must be someone else out here." Jody scanned a full three hundred and sixty degrees with his flashlight. "But we haven't been able to find him yet."

Denton's partner deflated the airbag and started to carefully remove Reed from the smashed SUV.

"Nothing obvious here," he told Denton. "Just a busted nose. He's moving everything and his breath sounds are good."

"Guys, over here." It was Jody's partner, his voice trembling, hollow.

It had come from the other side of the SUV, near the oak tree. Jody and Denton sloshed through a shallow ditch and headed in his direction.

Jody stopped, his feet frozen to the muddy ground. Denton almost ran into the paramedic, managed somehow to catch himself, and followed the beam of the officer's flashlight as it penetrated the darkness off to their right.

A barbed-wire fence, its bristling, rusted points wrapped around cedar posts and several small oak trees, lined the other side of the ditch. At the farthest reach of the flashlights, something was draped over the top strands of wire. Unmoving, its appendages suspended at awkward angles, it was at first unrecognizable—an amorphous, bloody—

"Case!"

Reed's cry disappeared into the muted darkness and the men sprang as one toward the fence.

"Still no pulse?"

Jeff Ryan had his fingers on Case Grissom's femoral artery. He shook his head. "Nothing."

I glanced up at the clock again. We had been working with this young man for almost an hour. The right side of his chest had been smashed when he was thrown from the SUV, and his right femur was broken. There had never been any sign of life at the scene, and we all knew the chances of his recovery were small, if not nonexistent. Yet he was only eighteen years old, and we were going to try.

Ten minutes later, I called it, and we all stepped back from the stretcher and the lifeless teenager.

"His parents are in the family room," Lori said quietly. "They want to see him."

She began to straighten the countertop and then moved to the stretcher. She hesitated for a moment, straightened his contorted leg, then placed a sheet over his broken body, pulling it to just under his chin.

"I'll go get them, if you're ready." She looked up at me and waited.

When are you ever ready for something like this? How do you prepare yourself for sharing this devastating news with total strangers?

"I think they know," Lori whispered as she turned and moved toward the door.

The Grissoms *did* know about their son, but it didn't make it any easier. I described his injuries, everything we had done for him, and that he didn't suffer. He was unconscious—gone—from the moment he flew out of the vehicle.

"If only he had been wearing his seat belt." His mother gently stroked his forehead. "How many times…"

Her voice trailed away, and her husband put his arm around her.

"Shh," was all he could say. It was enough.

I left them in major trauma with Lori and stepped over to the nurses' station.

Jody Bridges was writing his report and looked up as I walked over beside him.

"That's gotta be tough," he said, motioning with his head toward major trauma. "I still need to talk with them, when you think it's alright."

I nodded and stared at the countertop. It would never be alright.

"It's a bad stretch of road." Jody closed his notebook and leaned against the desk. "Especially when it's raining. There're a couple of spots where water pools on the pavement, right after you come out of that curve. I'm thinkin' they hydroplaned, spun out of control, and hit that big oak tree. That's when the Grissom boy was thrown out of the vehicle. Still can't believe the other kid wasn't hurt—at least not too bad. How is he, Doc?"

"He's going to be fine. His nose is broken and there's a big gash over it. One of the other doctors is sewing him up right now. But he didn't break anything else, and there's no head or neck injury. He was mighty lucky."

"You can say that again." The officer shifted his feet and rested an elbow on the countertop. "I'm still thinkin' that airbag saved him. The passenger bag might have helped the Grissom boy, but with the door torn off, I guess it blew him out of the SUV. It sure didn't stop him."

"Any alcohol involved?" Amy asked from behind the desk. That was a reasonable question, and all too often the case.

"Not a bit," Jody answered quickly. "Glad of that, for all of them. And no sign they were speeding, either. I think they just got unlucky, what with the rain and all. Wrong place, wrong time. It's a terrible thing."

The door of major trauma opened and I turned around. Lori was leading the Grissoms out of the room and quietly closed the door behind them. Mrs. Grissom stopped in the hallway and put a hand on the wooden door. Her head was bowed and she was sobbing. Jody Bridges cleared his throat and looked away.

"We're going back to the family room to make some calls." Lori's eyes caught mine and she gave me a small nod. I stood up straight, took a deep breath, and followed them.

We were halfway down the hall, just opposite the entrance to minor trauma. Lori walked on but the Grissoms stopped dead in their tracks. They were staring into the room and they both stiffened, their arms still around each other.

Reed Levin was lying on bed B in the back left corner of the room. One of my partners was bending over the stretcher, carefully placing some sutures in the open wound over his nose.

Reed's parents stood behind the stretcher, looking down at their son.

Silence. None of us moved. Slowly, as if he somehow knew we were standing in the hallway, Reed's father looked up at us. An instant later his mother followed his gaze.

Lori had turned around, and her eyes widened. She looked at the Grissoms and then at me. I shook my head, and we waited.

Anything could happen. I didn't know these people and couldn't begin to guess how they might respond, how they might react to the loss of their son while his friend—who had been driving the car—was alive, lying on a nearby stretcher.

Reed's mother looked into the eyes of Mrs. Grissom, and tears streamed down the cheeks of both women.

Painful seconds passed—then Mrs. Grissom walked over to the

stretcher and put her hand gently on Reed's shoulder. Slowly, without a word, his hands came up from the bed and grasped hers. He was sobbing, and his shudders shook the stretcher.

My partner stopped sewing, sat up straight, and looked down at Reed and then up at the woman standing beside him. He looked over at me and I nodded.

We stood there in silence, unmoving, for a few precious seconds—and the healing began.

Reed's parents stepped around the stretcher and stood beside Mrs. Grissom. Her husband walked over and the four looked at each other, tears flowing freely from every eye.

It was Mr. Grissom who moved first. His large, bearish arms reached out and pulled Mr. Levin to him. Then his wife grabbed Mrs. Levin and they all stood there together—a tangled, sobbing mass of grief and tears—and forgiveness.

The Frozen Snake

Lori Davidson burst through the triage entrance, her eyes wide and face flushed.

"Dr. Lesslie, you need to come look at this!"

A middle-aged man in a police uniform was holding a wad of bloody gauze to the left side of his neck. He sat slumped in the wheelchair Lori was pushing, and as they went by, Sergeant Mason Tolliver of the city police looked in my direction, caught my eye, and gave me a weak smile.

Lori wheeled him into major trauma and I dropped the chart in my hand to the countertop and darted after her.

We moved him to the stretcher and jacked the head of the bed to a sitting position. Lori whipped out a pair of large scissors from her dress pocket. She deftly separated his dark blue shirt, neatly swerving around his sergeant's badge. No time for undoing buttons.

"What happened?" I leaned close to the officer, checked the pulse in his left wrist, and carefully began to peel the layers of gauze from his neck.

"Something silly." He slowly shook his head a few times.

"Is he okay?" Through the doorway dashed a young policeman, Chad Brinkley. He had his partner's blood smeared on his hands and forearms. "Is he going to be alright?"

Brinkley's chest was heaving, and his pale face turned first to his partner and then to me.

"I'm going to be fine, Chad." Mason extended his right hand and the younger officer grabbed it.

"Let's take a look." I removed the last piece of gauze and glanced up at the overhead light. Lori stepped beside me, reached up, and adjusted the bright beam, focusing it on the gaping seven-inch wound. It extended from just below Mason's left ear to his collarbone. Blood was flowing from the edges of torn skin and muscle, but nothing was spurting—not yet.

Brinkley gasped and took a faltering step backward.

I saw movement in the doorway and looked over at Amy Connors. "What do you need, Dr. Lesslie?"

I glanced down at the wounded officer. Lori was starting an IV in his right arm and had several filled tubes of blood lying on the stretcher. "We'll need another IV," I said quietly to the nurse. Then to Amy, "We need lab stat, and a portable chest X-ray."

The secretary turned and I called after her, "And see who's on call for general surgery."

"Already done it." Harriet Gray slipped around the exiting Amy and stepped into the room. "Dr. Ravenel is upstairs making rounds and is headed this way."

"Thanks, Harriet." I nodded at her and turned back to Mason Tolliver. "Any other wounds that you know of, Sergeant?" He was now stripped from the waist up and I didn't see any other obvious injury.

"Nope, I think this is it." He tucked his chin to the left and smiled. "Probably enough, I suppose."

I heard shallow panting behind me. Lori quickly looked up and over my shoulder. Before I could turn around, Harriet had grabbed the arm of Officer Brinkley and guided him to a nearby chair.

"Have a seat, son," she told the pasty-white and sweating private. "Take a few slow, deep breaths. There, that's it."

"He's not used to this," Mason whispered. "It took him by surprise. Took *me* by surprise too."

"Who did this?" I leaned him forward a little, checking for any other wounds of his upper back.

He sighed heavily and shook his head. "Freddy Parsons."

Lori's head jerked up and her eyes sought mine.

From behind me I heard Harriet's "hmm-hmm," and the sixty-year-old nurse stepped over to the stretcher.

She put her hands on the rail and looked down at Mason. "Freddy Parsons." Her words were slow, deliberate, and they hung heavily in the air above his bed.

Trying to get a good look at Mason's entire back, I twisted around him and saw the one-inch circular scar—still purplish and angry.

"The same Freddy Parsons who shot you in the back ten years ago?" This time Harriet's voice was a low rumble. "I thought he was in prison."

Sergeant Mason Tolliver and his partner, Danny Childs, were responding to an altercation on Dutchman Street. "Gunshots fired," the dispatcher had warned.

It was midnight, the middle of winter, and the two officers were the first at the scene.

Mason looked at the younger officer and noticed his incessant lip-licking. "First time?"

Danny kept staring at the ramshackle house in front of them and nodded—and licked his lips.

"That's okay." Mason reached out and put a firm hand on Childs's shoulder. "Just let me take the lead on this one."

They slowly approached the sad clapboard dwelling and were halfway up the cracked cement sidewalk, when the rickety screen door flew open. They froze, pointing their weapons, as two teenage boys bolted out the door, glanced once in their direction, and hightailed it for the nearby woods.

Danny took a step in their direction and Mason grabbed his elbow. "Nope, not them. We're going inside."

The screen door was bravely hanging by one twisted, rusted hinge, and almost fell off when Mason moved it aside. The officers stepped into what could once have been a comfortable living room. Now it was only dank, dark, and depressing. A single lightbulb hung from the ceiling, splashing shadows on a couple of worn chairs and a tattered, blue sofa. The young man sitting on the sofa looked up as the officers approached, his eyes glazed from some illicit medication, his brain absent.

"Put your hands on your head!" Danny called out. When the man didn't respond, he repeated his order, louder this time. Still no response.

Danny was moving toward the sofa, when the gunshot exploded in his ears. A burning sensation tore through his left hand and up his arm. He spun to his left, just as Mason fell awkwardly to the floor and a sickening *thump* echoed through the cold, gloomy room.

Freddy Parsons sat in a dilapidated wooden chair, its wobbly legs straining to hold his weight. He was holding a .38 in his hand, pointing it at the fallen police officer.

Later, after the adrenaline cleared his brain and he could think clearly, Danny tried to remember what happened next.

"I don't know why I didn't shoot the guy right then and there. I was squeezing down on the trigger, bracing myself for the shot, and the man looked at me and tossed the gun on the floor. Then he put his hands up in the air and sat there, grinning."

The slug from Freddy Parsons' .38 had passed through Danny's left hand before hitting Mason in his back. The sergeant had surgery that night and recovered without any complications. Danny Childs resigned from the police force and moved from Rock Hill with his wife and two small children. Freddy Parsons went to prison.

While in the "big house" in Columbia, Freddy had been visited by Mason Tolliver. At first Freddy wouldn't utter a word. Over time the two developed a kind of relationship—not quite a friendship—but they began to talk with each other.

Freddy behaved, studied some automotive repair books, and was going to "make a new start" when he got out of prison. Mason encouraged the younger man and advised him to keep his nose clean. The officer continued his visits every couple of months until Freddy was finally released. "Good behavior," the report had read. "Good chance of becoming a productive member of society."

—————

"So it *was* Freddy Parsons who did this to you." Harriet stepped over to the stretcher and put a hand on Mason's shoulder. "How did *this* happen?"

The chair behind us grated roughly across the floor and officer Chad Brinkley rose slowly to his feet. "I'll tell you how it happened, Mrs. Gray. Sarge and I were responding to an altercation and were the first unit to arrive. We walked into this beat-up house on Dutchman and found this guy—Freddy Parsons—sitting on a coffee table. Sarge knew him and they started talking. Seemed like friends and all."

I glanced down at Mason. His eyes were closed, squeezed shut as if his partner's words were arrows.

"Everything seemed calm," Chad continued. "Then all of a sudden these two guys busted out of the back room and headed for the front door. I grabbed my weapon and was about to holler for them to stop, when Freddy jumped up with this huge knife and slashed Sarge's throat. Blood was flying everywhere—they were all out the door before I could do anything. I ripped off part of my shirt and held it over his neck till the EMS got there."

"Thanks again, Chad." Mason's eyes were open once more, and he was looking at the young policeman.

Harriet squeezed Mason's shoulder. "A frozen snake." She looked down at the sergeant and smiled.

With eyebrows raised, he stared up at the nurse and slowly shook his head.

"Let me explain." Harriet shifted her feet and settled against the stretcher rail. "The story goes like this—there was this man, about your age I think, and he was walking to town one day. There had been a terrible blizzard and snow was everywhere. It was freezing. The man could barely see to take one step in front of the other, but all of a sudden, he saw a snake lying in the middle of the road—frozen solid. He stopped, bent over, and picked up that snake—stiff as a stick. Now you need to understand something about this man—he was kindhearted and didn't like to see anything or anyone suffer. So he opened up his jacket and tucked that snake up against his neck, trying to warm it up.

"After a couple of miles, he felt the snake begin to move a little, to wriggle around. Then out of nowhere, the snake bit him! Right on the neck! The man reached down, grabbed the snake, and held it in front of him. 'Why did you bite me?' he demanded. 'I rescued you from the frozen road and warmed you—I brought you back to life.' Well, the snake just looked at the man all beady-eyed and finally said, 'You knew I was a snake when you picked me up.'"

The room was silent. Harriet raised her eyebrows, looked down at Sergeant Tolliver, and slowly nodded. "Mason, you *knew* Freddy Parsons was a snake."

The police officer didn't say anything for a moment—he just lay there.

Finally he looked up at the grandmotherly nurse, and a smile slowly spread across his face.

> *Peter came to Jesus and asked,*
> *"Lord, how many times shall I forgive my brother*
> *or sister who sins against me?*
> *Up to seven times?"*
> *Jesus answered, "I tell you,*
> *Not seven times, but seventy-seven times."*
> Matthew 18:21-22

THE *Miracle*
OF HUMILITY

*All those who exalt themselves
will be humbled,
and those who humble themselves
will be exalted.*

JESUS, in Luke 14:11

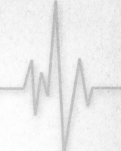

Step Aside

The door to major trauma flew open and Grayson Peerman stormed into the room.

"Okay, what have we got here? Heard there was a stab wound."

Grayson was one of the general surgeons on staff—not one of our favorites. He was known for his short temper, arrogance, and unwarranted outbursts. He was wearing a sweat-stained surgical cap, scrubs, and blood-spattered shoe covers. He must have just come from the OR. I looked over at Lori Davidson and shook my head.

In three giant strides, he was beside the stretcher, staring down at our newly arrived patient, TC. TC had just been brought in by EMS after an altercation somewhere downtown, and we didn't have a last name yet. He had been stabbed in the belly and left on the sidewalk. He was awake, but his blood pressure was low and his skin was pale and pasty.

I had just stepped into the room myself and Lori was starting an IV. The two paramedics were gathering their equipment and trying to leave as fast as they could. We all knew Dr. Grayson Peerman.

The surgeon placed his huge hand on TC's abdomen and began prodding around the injury, which was located four or five inches above his belly button. Then with no glove and no warning he probed the wound with his index finger, his head tilted to one side while he stared at the ceiling.

TC objected, or so his string of profanity would lead us to believe.

"Calm down, son," Peerman chastised him. "If I'm going to save your life, I need to know what I'm dealing with."

Peerman withdrew his bloody finger and wiped it on the stretcher sheet.

"I'm on call and was passing through the ER. I'll take over now. When's the last time he ate?" He glanced over at Lori.

She flushed and stammered, "We haven't had time to—"

Peerman silenced her with an opened palm, then looked down at TC. "When's the last time you had something to eat?" he asked loudly, as if the young man must be hard of hearing.

TC shook his head and held his abdomen. "I don't remember. Maybe—"

"Doesn't matter," Peerman waved his hand and turned to Lori. "Get some routine labs and type and cross for four units. Then call the OR and tell them what we've got. And turn his IV up, wide open. Got that?"

"Yes, Doctor," Lori answered. She walked over to the phone sitting on the countertop. "Do you want a chest X-ray, Dr. Peerman? His breath sounds on the left side are diminished and he was stabbed by a *man.* He might have—"

"Don't have time. It's a stab wound, young lady—of the abdomen. And it doesn't matter if he was stabbed by a man or a woman or a monkey. He sounds fine to me."

My heard jerked around at this. *When had he listened to this guy's chest?*

The surgeon turned to the stretcher, held out his hand for Lori's stethoscope, then placed it on TC's chest—first the right side, then the left, and finally over his abdomen.

"Sounds fine to me." He tossed the stethoscope onto the stretcher and walked out of the room.

I looked at Lori and reached for the stethoscope draped over my left shoulder. The radio of one of the paramedics sounded its alarm just as I was bending over to listen to TC's chest.

"This is EMS 3. We're at the back door with a twenty-three-year-old unknown overdose. Unresponsive."

"You'd better go." Lori nodded at the door then picked up the phone. "I'll call the OR."

I was opening the door when she added, "And Dr. Lesslie, I *do* pay attention to you sometimes."

I chuckled but didn't turn around. I knew what she was talking about. She remembered a comment I had made—maybe a couple of years ago— about the difference between how a woman stabs someone and how a man does it. A woman will usually grab the handle and stab downward, while a man will poke the blade into his victim. If TC's assailant had been a man and they had both been standing, that poke could have been aimed upward and pierced his diaphragm and then his lung. If it collapsed—

The ambulance doors opened and EMS wheeled their OD patient into the department.

"Cardiac?" the paramedic asked me.

"Yeah," I answered. "Let's go."

A few minutes later, I stepped into the hallway, looking for Amy Connors. Grayson Peerman was still standing at the nurses' station, writing on some scattered pieces of paper. We both heard the mechanized rumbling of the portable X-ray machine as it rolled down the hallway and turned into major trauma.

"Hold on there!" he shouted at the two young techs. "What's going on? I didn't order a chest X-ray."

He stomped over to where they stood and leaned into their flushing faces.

"Who ordered this?"

"The anesthesiologist said—" The X-ray tech was frightened, whispering, and I could barely hear what she was saying.

"Speak up, young lady!" Peerman's nose was only inches from the young woman's.

"The anesthesiologist said the patient needed a chest X-ray!" she blurted, looking down at the floor and backing into the machine. "He said he wouldn't put him to sleep without one."

"Why that…" Peerman's face was beet-red and he was spraying spit everywhere. He looked from side to side and finally said, "Do what he says. I'll deal with this later."

He spun around and stalked back to the nurses' station. I nodded at the techs and they wheeled the machine into trauma, glancing over their shoulders a couple of times before disappearing into the room.

Our OD patient was stable, and I was at the nurses' station when one of the X-ray techs returned with TC's chest films. They slid them onto the countertop, glanced at Dr. Peerman, and scurried back down the hallway. Out of the corner of my eye I could see his head tilt down toward the X-ray folder and then quickly snap away.

The phone rang and Amy picked it up.

"Okay, I'll let him know."

She hung up the receiver and looked up at Peerman. "They're ready for your patient in the OR, Doctor."

"Hmm," he muttered, and didn't look up.

I picked up the X-ray folder and walked across the hallway to trauma. The door was open and I stepped in, turned to the view box, and snapped the film into place.

"Well, would you look at that." I glanced over my shoulder and beckoned Lori with a nod.

"What is it?" She walked over behind me and stared at the X-ray. I didn't say anything, but just waited.

"Oh," was all she said. Her right index went to the view box and traced the edge of his collapsed left lung. It was down by at least 50 percent.

"You were right, Lori. This would have been a disaster."

"Right about what?" Grayson Peerman was standing in the doorway, scowling, his clenched fists on his hips.

I looked over at Lori and raised my eyebrows. "Your turn," I whispered.

"Right about what?" Peerman repeated, louder and more agitated this time.

This was a great opportunity for Lori to educate this obnoxious, overbearing man. If ever there was a time to say, "I told you so," this was it.

I cleared my throat and stepped around Peerman and out into the hallway. I stopped just out of sight and listened.

"Dr. Peerman, you might want to look at this." That was all she said. As she walked out of the room, she caught my eye and winked.

That was it? "You might want to look at this"? This was her big chance!

But then, this was Lori Davidson.

Suddenly from inside the trauma room: "What th——!"

The Teeth of the Dragon

The metal basin clattered down the hallway, and everyone in the department jerked their heads toward the doorway of major trauma. Wait... wait...there it was—another shiny object sailed through the door, ricocheted off a stainless-steel supply cart, and clanged loudly before coming to rest against the far wall. It was only a matter of time—moments—before the dragon would appear.

And there he was. Edward Morgan burst through the doorway and into the hall. He stood there, fists on hips, feet wide apart, face flushed to a fire-engine red. If it were physically possible, steam would be escaping his ears. He was the picture of—of—Edward Morgan.

Morgan was one of three neurosurgeons on the medical staff of the hospital and had the well-earned reputation of having a hair-trigger temper, total disregard for anyone other than himself, and a proclivity for causing the biggest disturbance possible. (Hence the metal pans scattered in the hallway.)

"I need some help in here!"

It wasn't a calm, quiet request. His angry scream quickly grabbed the attention of everyone in the ER, including nearly all of the patients. Those who were able were peeking around curtains, eyes large, mouths hanging open. For those of us who knew Edward Morgan, it was just another day at the office.

I looked down at Amy Connors. "I thought someone was back there with him."

She kept her nose in the logbook and slowly shook her head. Finally she looked up at me. "Angie Davis was assigned major trauma, and I thought—"

Her words hung in the air. She was staring down the hall in the direction of Dr. Morgan. I turned just in time to see Angie slip out of trauma and scurry toward the back of the department. Her cheeks were a fiery red and she was dabbing one of her eyes with Kleenex.

She didn't escape the attention of Morgan. He glanced over his shoulder, pointed at her with an angry index finger, then glowered in my direction.

"I need some *competent* help! And I need it right now!"

He stomped back into major trauma and slammed the door.

"Man, where is Virginia Granger when you need her?" Amy shook her head again and once more buried herself in the logbook.

Virginia, our head nurse, was on vacation this week. But I wasn't sure she would be able to do any good with a ballistic Edward Morgan. She had tried in the past to calm him down. We all had—even the administration—but the outcome was always the same. He might get quiet for a few minutes, but then something else would set him off and he would explode.

Like the time with the telephone.

We had called him about a young man involved in an auto accident—possible neck injury. We needed him to take a look at the guy. He hadn't been exactly pleasant on the phone, and by the time he got to the ER he was pretty fired up.

"Drunk, I bet."

The huffy accusation had been rhetorical, but I made the mistake of picking it up.

"Actually not, Edward. He was driving home from work and hit a patch of ice. Slipped off the road and into a ditch. No alcohol involved."

He jerked around and speared me with a piercing stare.

"Careless, then. Just careless."

I smiled at him and turned away.

"Get me the radiologist on the phone." It was a demand, not a request.

Amy reached for the receiver but Morgan was quicker.

"Never mind, I'll do it."

He dialed the extension for radiology—8242. No answer, silence. He dialed again—the same thing. Silence.

Amy must have noticed that he hadn't punched 9 before dialing the extension.

"Dr. Morgan—"

"What th—!"

He snatched the phone from the desktop and ripped the cord and face plate from the wall, scattering pieces of Sheetrock around the nurses' station. Not satisfied with this level of destruction, he heaved the phone at a nearby trash can, knocking it over and spilling its contents across the floor.

"Never mind! I'll go over there myself!"

He snorted and grumbled down the hallway and out of the department.

"Amy, shouldn't we call X-ray and warn them?"

"With what?"

And then there was the time Virginia refused to call the administration and complain about the lack of an operating room for one of his patients. Morgan had a simple elective procedure to do, and all of the ORs were occupied with emergency cases.

"Dr. Morgan, I've called the OR supervisor," Virginia explained for the third time. "And they will call us as soon as one of the rooms is available."

"And just what am I supposed to do? Just sit over here and wait?"

Amy shifted in her seat and quietly slid her phone out of view.

Morgan began pacing in front of the nurses' station, mumbling something I couldn't understand.

He walked over to the ambulance entrance and stopped before stepping onto the mat that opened the automatic door. He turned to his right, reached out, and grabbed the fire extinguisher.

Amy ducked, and Virginia Granger called out, "Dr. Morgan!"

Too late. He tore the red cylinder off the wall and with surprising ease, slung it down the ER hallway. Fortunately, no one was struck. But the discharge mechanism was somehow activated and a white cloud spread through the department.

Virginia stared at the billowing mess. Her jaw hardened, and with narrowed eyes she turned and stalked toward the miscreant neurosurgeon.

He was gone—he'd disappeared through the ambulance entrance and into the night.

"So, who's gonna go help him?" Amy tilted her head in the direction of major trauma. The door was still closed, and no one was rushing to open it.

"What's he got in there? I didn't call him for anything."

"I think it's a dressing change on one of his rehab patients." She paused and searched her desk for the clipboard of major trauma. "I think the guy was in the hospital and Dr. Morgan brought him down here. Didn't call or anything. You know how he is."

We *all* knew how he was. I needed to go check on Angie Davis and, as much as I didn't want to, I would stick my head in trauma on the way.

"I'll go help him."

Amy and I jerked around as Margie Suttles walked up to the counter.

"I'll go help Dr. Morgan," she repeated.

Amy's eyes were wide. "Are you sure, Margie? That's Dr. Morgan. *The* Dr. Morgan."

"I know who he is." Her voice was calm, quiet. "I'll go help him."

Margie was a new graduate nurse and had only been in the department for a few months. She was still technically "orienting" and hadn't yet been given a solo assignment. She was young, composed, soft-spoken, and assured. And we were about to send her into the very teeth of the dragon.

"Margie, I—"

"I can handle this, Dr. Lesslie."

Margie walked around the nurses' station and over to the door of major trauma. She hesitated, but only for an instant. The door gave way to her push, then closed behind her.

Before I could say a word, Amy reached down, flipped on the intercom for major trauma, and held an index finger to her lips. I leaned as far over the counter as I could and listened.

"I said I needed some *competent* help." Morgan's voice was still belligerent but not as loud. "And just who are *you*, young lady? Obviously no one possessing any competence."

"I'm Margie Suttles, one of the nurses on the ER staff. And I'm here to—"

"Don't waste your time. You can—"

"Dr. Morgan, stop right there."

Amy and I stared at each other, our mouths open.

"I am perfectly capable of helping you with this patient." Her words were calm, measured. "And I think I need to tell you what my grandmother has often told me. 'You'll catch a lot more flies with honey than with vinegar.'"

Amy shook her head and drew her hand across her neck, knifelike.

We waited for the explosion.

"What are you trying to say, young lady?"

This was no explosion. The tone of Morgan's voice was one of surprise. He sounded like he might really want the answer to this question.

"It's just that we're all trying to do the same thing—take care of our patients. And when we're all a little nicer, things go better."

A foreboding silence.

We braced ourselves for the clang of flying metal pans.

Instead, there was a quiet "hmm." Then, "Ms. Suttles, let me show you how we need to do this."

Amy flipped off the intercom and we looked at each other, speechless.

A few minutes later, the door of major trauma opened. Dr. Edward Morgan stepped into the hallway, cleared his throat, and turned in our direction. He hitched up his pants, cocked his head, and uttered a faint "hmm."

There was no smile on his face. But there wasn't a scowl, either. Then he was gone.

Margie stepped through the doorway, a bundle of bandages in her hands. We were staring at her with wide eyes and slack jaws.

She glanced over at us and halted in the hallway. She looked from Amy to me then back to Amy. Finally she shrugged.

"What?"

The Dragon Slayer, and she didn't even know it.

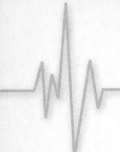

Coming Home to Roost

"Dr. Lesslie, let me tell you how this is going to work."

Bill Corley stood in front of me, his thick-rimmed glasses riding low on his long, bulbous nose. His arms were folded across his chest, just below some intricate embroidery:

Dr. William Corley, MD
Specialist in Internal Medicine

The ER was hopping, and I had taken a few precious moments to meet Rich Aberman's new partner.

Corley stared at me, and when I didn't say anything, he repeated himself. "Let me tell you how this is going to work."

I glanced over at Rich and raised my eyebrows. He quickly lowered his head and looked away. I was on my own.

"Okay, Bill, exactly what do you mean?"

"It's *Dr. Corley*." He stiffened and his right foot started to tap. "I expect to be addressed as that when I receive calls from the emergency department."

Rich cleared his throat and raised a hesitant hand to his chin.

"Fine." I nodded and reached for a chart on the countertop. We were standing in front of the nurses' station, and I suspected that Amy Connors was enjoying all of this.

"I'll be sure to tell—"

"Once again," Corley interrupted. "Let me tell you how this is going to work. I've spent a lot of time in various ERs and I understand how you and your staff *dump* on other physicians. Well, let me make it perfectly clear—you will *not* dump on me. Do I need to repeat myself?"

Rich looked up and in a quiet voice said, "Bill, I think that once you get to know—"

Corley's eyes continued to bore into mine. "Is that clear?"

I tossed the chart in my hand onto the counter. The clipboard clattered loudly a few times before coming to rest in front of Amy. She glanced up at me with eyebrows raised. Her elbows found the desktop and she cradled her head in her hands, her eyes moving from me to Corley, and back to me.

"Bill...*Dr.* Corley. Rich tells me that you've been in the military since finishing medical school. I'm sure you are well-trained, but your military emergency departments must work a little differently than all the others in the country. It's not the *medical* staff of a hospital that gets 'dumped on,' as you put it. It's those of us in the ER. We're the last line, the bottom of the rung. When you're tired or in bed, *we're* the ones you send your patients to. And we're glad to see them. All we ask is that you respond when we ask for your help. *That's* how things work around here."

My face was flushed and my heart was hammering in my chest. I had said enough.

"Bill." Rich stepped forward a little, almost between Corley and me. "Dr. Lesslie and his team are great to work with. You'll see. I just wanted you to meet him and—"

"We'll see," Corley fumed. "But understand me—I will *not* be dumped on."

He spun around and stomped down the hallway. Rich shrugged, gave me a feeble smile, and hurried after his younger partner.

I stood there shaking my head, trying to calm down.

"Looks like *you've* made a friend." Amy snickered and slid the abused chart across the counter. "Boy, Dr. Aberman is such a nice guy, and all his patients love him. Why in the world would he bring on somebody like Genghis Khan—what's his name? Bill Ketchup?"

"Bill Corley," I mumbled. "And I don't know why. Maybe Rich sees something in this man that isn't readily apparent. Maybe he's great with his patients but has trouble interacting with...us..." I paused, struggling to find the right word.

"Us *lowlifes*?" Amy chuckled and pushed her chair back. "You really think someone who acts like that is good to his patients?"

―――――

He wasn't. Dr. William Corley quickly made a name for himself with the entire staff of the emergency department. When called about one of his patients, he was rude, blunt, sometimes abusive. And when he reluctantly arrived in the ER, his displeasure was plainly engraved on his face and in his eyes.

"He's not a very happy person," Virginia Granger had profoundly pronounced one morning. "Some people just carry a dark cloud with them. Some of them—maybe Dr. Corley included—seem to enjoy it."

Mattie Caufman was the next to find herself in Corley's dark and cloudy shadow. Her daughter, Brenda Mayes, had brought the ninety-two-year-old Mattie to the ER one Sunday morning because of cough, fever, and shortness of breath.

I pulled the curtain of room 5 to one side and stepped over to the stretcher.

"Mattie, what have you been up to *this* time?" We had seen this cheerful, animated nonagenarian several times in the ER, usually with minor problems—a sprained wrist suffered while playing tetherball with a great-granddaughter, a hand burned while baking Christmas cookies, and most recently a cut finger from slicing onions for a family picnic.

It wasn't minor this time. Mattie was sick.

She managed a weak smile and a weaker wave of her slender hand.

"Not so good this morning, Dr. Lesslie. I think I may have pneumonia." Her voice was faint and her respirations labored.

"Let's just find out about that." I looked again at her clipboard.

Temp—103.2
Respirations—20
HR—108
BP—92/60

Brenda got up from the chair in the corner of the room and walked over beside me. "Momma started to get sick yesterday. She didn't want to come to the ER—didn't want to be a nuisance—but when she was too short of breath to walk to the kitchen, she decided it was time."

Mattie shook her head. "I don't want to be a burden."

"Mattie, you're never a burden," I told her. "That's why we're here—to get you back on that tetherball court with your granddaughter."

"*Great*-granddaughter," she corrected me. "And I've had to give that up, after the wrist injury and all."

Her blood work came back with a sky-high white count and low sodium—both red flags for real problems. She was right about the pneumonia. Her X-ray showed a completely socked-in right-lower lobe. She was going to be in the hospital for several days, probably starting off in the ICU.

"Amy, who's on call for Dr. Aberman?" His name had been written on Mattie's chart under "Family MD."

"You don't want to know." Amy frowned, shook her head, and punched some numbers on her phone.

"You're kidding? Corley?"

"That's right." She handed me the receiver. "Genghis himself."

I took the phone, placed it to my ear, and waited.

"What is it?" Corley's voice finally grumbled, sending warm and fuzzy feelings all through me.

I explained Mattie's troubles and that she would need to be admitted to the hospital.

"*I'll* decide that issue." Click.

Warm and fuzzy.

Thirty minutes later, I was standing in front of Amy, just outside room 5. Moments earlier, Bill Corley had snatched Mattie Caufman's chart from the countertop and stomped into the room, snapping the curtain closed behind him.

"And just *why* are you in the ER today?" he demanded.

His voice carried through most of the department, and Amy looked up at me and shook her head.

"Why...I..." was the feeble reply.

"Speak up! I have other patients to attend. I repeat—why are you in the ER today?"

This went on for several minutes, time enough for me to put a stop to it. I turned, took a step, and was nearly bowled over when a red-faced Corley stormed out of the room. He never addressed me or looked in my direction, but walked over to the counter and flung the chart on Amy's desk, narrowly missing her hand.

"Find a bed in the ICU and call me when she's upstairs."

Corley spun around and stalked down the hallway, his dark cloud straining to keep pace.

"One of these days..." Amy grumbled.

I pulled the curtain aside and stepped into room 5. Brenda Mayes was standing in the corner clutching the back of her neck, tears streaming down her reddened cheeks.

"Mrs. Mayes, Mattie, I'm sorry about—"

"Tsk, tsk," Mattie clucked, smiling up at me. "You don't have anything to be sorry about. But that Dr. Corley—he certainly is an angry young man, isn't he?"

We talked for a while and I explained what would happen with Mattie in the ICU. I tried to calm Brenda, but she remained upset and angry. Mattie was fine.

"You know, Dr. Lesslie," she whispered between difficult breaths. "Sometimes these things, just like chickens, come home to roost." She paused and looked at the closed curtain. "I'm afraid your Dr. Corley is going to have to learn that lesson."

Three weeks later, Dr. William Corley's chickens came home to roost. Rich Aberman terminated his employment with the group, and Corley was gone. We never saw him again in the ER. Rich told me he was somewhere in Oklahoma but wasn't practicing medicine.

Months later, Rich was seeing one of his patients in the ER and told me he had recently talked with Bill Corley.

"Robert, he sounded like a completely different person. He's joined an internal-medicine group and seems to be completely happy. And he said something that almost knocked me down. He said he was really *enjoying* his patients. Can you believe that?"

I *could* believe it, after recently bumping into Brenda Mayes during a concert at Winthrop University. Mattie was at home recuperating from her pneumonia, and her daughter and I had a chance to talk about that Sunday morning in the ER.

"God bless Momma." Brenda shook her head and glanced at the distant ceiling. "She just sat there and smiled while that doctor went on and on. *I* was the one getting upset—but I suppose you saw that. I couldn't speak, I was so mad. When he finally stopped yelling at us, Momma motioned for him to come close to her stretcher and she whispered something. I had to strain to hear, but I did. She told him that to walk with the Lord, to really get to know him, you have to be humble. A proud man has only himself for company, and that's a long and lonely journey. Then she looked him right in the eye and said, 'Doctor, I hope your journey isn't lonely.' He didn't say another word—just walked out of the room."

"*Enjoying* his patients," Rich repeated. "Can you believe it? What do you suppose got into him?"

Yes, I *did* believe it. And it wasn't *what*—it was *Who.*

THE *Miracle* OF...
COINCIDENCE

*Coincidence is the word we use
when we can't see the levers and pulleys.*

EMMA BULL (1954–)

Expect the Unexpected

There, right in front of me, was the answer. But it wasn't what I expected.

Toby Meyers, a precocious, active three-year-old boy, had been brought to the ER by his mother. For the past week or so he had been coughing, running high temps, and occasionally wheezing. No history of asthma and no medical problems. Prior to this, he had been the picture of health and, I'm sure, quite a handful.

"We took him to a clinic down at the beach last weekend," his mother had explained. "Same thing—cough, fever. They told us he had bronchitis and to take this." She reached into her oversized purse and took out a bottle of liquid medicine with pink smears down its side. Amoxicillin. "He's no better, and still coughs a lot. Mainly at night."

Toby looked up at me, smiled, and coughed twice. "See?" he said, then coughed twice more.

His temperature was 102.2 and I heard noises on the right side of his chest. If he had had bronchitis last weekend, there was a good chance it was now pneumonia.

"We need to get an X-ray of his chest," I told his mother. "Just to be sure it's not pneumonia."

"What's 'moanya'?" he asked, looking first at his mother and then at me.

"Don't worry, Toby. I'm sure Dr. Lesslie is going to get you feeling better."

Now, here before me on the view box, was the answer. Toby did in fact have a right-sided pneumonia. But there was something else on the X-ray. Somewhere in his right lower lobe was a small, round metallic object—the size of a BB. It was just above the pneumonia, and would explain why the infection had developed in a perfectly healthy child. This wouldn't be a simple "change up the medicine and get well in a couple of days." Whatever this was would need to come out.

I walked back into his room and held up the X-ray for his mother to see.

"What is that?" she asked, immediately pointing to the round object.

"It looks like a BB to me," I explained. "Any chance he could have been playing with some and gotten them into his mouth?"

"A BB?" She spun around and stared at her son. "Toby, have you been playing with some BBs? Did you swallow one?"

Toby's face flushed and he looked at his mother and then at me. "No, I didn't play with any BBs," he muttered. His head dropped to his chest and his eyes found the floor. "Johnny, he made me do it. He dared me to eat some of them, and I…I'm sorry, Momma."

It turned out that Johnny was Toby's older brother. Mystery solved. I explained to their mother what would need to happen and walked out of the room and over to the nurses' station. Jason Wood, the other ER doc on duty with me that day, was standing there writing on a chart.

He glanced over as I dropped Toby's X-ray onto the countertop.

"What you got there?" He picked up the film and held it up to a ceiling light. "Wow, what do you think that is, other than a pneumonia?"

"Looks like a BB to me." Amy Connors was sitting behind the counter, straining her neck to see the film. She leaned back in her chair and looked at me. "Whatcha think? Did the kid aspirate a BB? Or did he get shot?"

"A BB!" Jason pointed at the foreign body. "You're right, Amy. That's what it looks like."

I told them Toby's story, and of my surprise when I saw the X-ray.

"You just never know, Robert," Jason said. "It's like Amy always says, you gotta expect the unexpected in the ER."

He dropped the X-ray back on the counter and slid his chart back in front of him. With pen poised in midair he looked over at me and said, "That reminds me of a patient I saw during my residency."

"Oh boy, here we go." Amy shook her head and shuffled the stack of papers on her desk. "Another one of your tall tales I bet." Jason was known to tell some stories, all of which he swore were true. "And I bet it's gonna start with 'It was a dark and stormy night…'"

Jason looked down at the secretary and smiled. "As a matter of fact, it *was* a dark and stormy night. I was a resident at Charlotte Memorial, and Dirk Trueblood—I'll never forget his name—came walking into the ER."

It was a little after midnight, and the triage nurse led the twenty-eight-year-old Dirk into one of the treatment rooms. She walked over to the nurses' station and handed the chart to Jason. "Fell over a chair and thinks he cracked some ribs. Pretty sore, but he looks okay."

Jason walked into the exam room and pulled up a chair. "So, you think you might have broken some ribs. Tell me what happened."

Dirk Trueblood proceeded to explain the reason for his late-night visit to the ER. He was putting his young boy to bed, flipped off the light, slipped on a carpet, and fell over a wooden chair. The chair back had caught him on his right chest and knocked the breath out of him. His lungs sounded okay, but he was really tender over his right ribs and was already starting to bruise. Jason sent him around to radiology for some X-rays of his chest.

It was an hour later when the tech brought Dirk back to the department. Without a word, she dropped his films on the counter and disappeared.

"Would you look at that," Jason muttered to himself, peering closely at the X-rays now on the view box. "How in the world…"

Dirk didn't have any obvious fractured ribs, and his underlying lung looked okay. But there was something else there. Something unexpected.

Jason walked back into the exam room and over to Mr. Trueblood. "Have you ever had any chest problems before, or been in some kind of altercation?"

"Altercation? What do you mean?"

"A fight, or some kind of assault."

Dirk scratched his chin and stared at the tiled floor. He shook his head, then suddenly dropped his hand and looked up at Jason. "About five years ago, I was brought in here with a cut on my arm." He rolled up his right arm sleeve, revealing a jagged ten-inch scar. "Somebody here stitched me up, but I don't remember very much. I had been at a friend's and probably had too much to drink. It was the next morning, when I sobered up, that I realized what had happened." He rolled his sleeve down and shook his head. "I was a little wilder back then."

"Anything else happen that night? Or have you had any other occasions when you…had too much to drink and got hurt?"

"No, that was it. Why?"

"Well, something is showing up on your X-ray, and— Have you had any neck problems? Any pain or maybe some numbness in your arm or hand?"

Dirk reached up and rubbed the back of his neck. "No. No neck pain. But now that you mention it, I've had some numbness in these two fingers for a couple of weeks." He held up his left hand and pointed to his long and ring fingers. "Seems to be getting worse. But what does that have to do with my neck?"

Jason walked around behind him and examined the back of his neck, just below his hairline.

There it was. A faint, thin scar, about three quarters of an inch long. He pressed down on the scar and the area around it. "Does that hurt, Mr. Trueblood?"

"No, it doesn't hurt, Doc. But when you press down, I can feel that numbness in my fingers. Weird." He shook his hand a couple of times then looked up at Jason. "What does that mean?"

"Let's go look at your X-rays."

One of the views of Dirk's chest revealed most of his neck as well. There, lying neatly between two of the vertebrae, was a four-inch pointed object aimed directly at his spinal cord. A knife blade.

～～～

"That thing must have been sitting in his neck for five years," Jason said, looking first at me and then down at Amy. "He didn't even know it. Whoever slashed his arm must have meant business and stabbed him in the neck—and the blade broke off. Within a couple of hours, we had him in the OR having it taken out. It must have been moving, getting closer to his spinal cord. The neurosurgeon said it was one, maybe two millimeters away. A funny movement or simple fall and that knife blade could have pithed him, paralyzed him completely. He was one lucky guy."

"He was lucky he fell over that chair," I said. "And he was lucky he came to the ER and saw you."

"See, it's like I said," Amy pronounced, rolling back in her chair. "In the ER, you've got to always expect the unexpected."

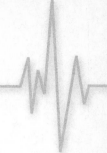

All That Glitters

Wednesday, 2:35 a.m. In the ER, we're always happy—thankful—for a straightforward diagnosis. Give us something simple we can deal with, something uncomplicated we can treat. It doesn't happen very often, but when it does, it is appreciated. Sometimes that simple, uncomplicated diagnosis is made the moment a patient walks into the department, but then...it's the ER.

"We're headed to ENT." Jeff Ryan was leading a young woman through triage, and the two paused at the nurses' station for a brief instant. But it was enough.

Maylee Strait was twenty-seven years old, probably five-foot-five, and weighed at least three hundred pounds. She was wearing a light-blue bathrobe that barely met in the front and large pink curlers adorning the top of her head. An older woman appeared behind her, and I assumed it was her mother.

Maylee looked over the counter and gave me a beaming smile. Suddenly her eyes widened and her mouth dropped open. She took in a huge breath, and I reached to cover my ears. Too late.

"Aaaahhh!"

The blood-curdling scream echoed off the walls of the ER and down the hall. Every head in the department turned in Maylee's direction. Her hands flew up in the air, covered her ears, and she started to dance. Not really dance—it was more of a gyration, a spasmodic jerking and tilting from one side to the other. She spun around a few times, almost sending Jeff flying into the far wall, and finally came to a sudden halt, staring right into my eyes.

"Help me, Mister! Help me!"

Before Jeff could reach out and steady the young woman, she had completely calmed herself. Her hands dropped to her side, she vigorously shook her head a couple of times, and that huge smile spread once again over her face.

I looked up at Jeff and nodded. "ENT. One of us will be right there."

Jeff led Maylee down the hall but her mother lingered a moment, watching her daughter as she shuffled down the hallway and disappeared into the ear, nose, and throat room.

She stepped over to the counter, smoothed her hair, cleared her throat, and—

"Aaaahhh!"

The scream reverberated again through the department and I couldn't help but flinch.

"What do you think's wrong with her? You don't seem too worried."

Frank Dixon was sitting beside me, looking a bit puzzled. He had been working in the ER as an MD for a little over three months and was well-trained, confident, easygoing, but still a little green. This would be a good teaching moment.

"When Jeff brings the chart back, why don't you go take a look?" I leaned back in my chair, folded my hands behind my head, and added, "Let me know what you think."

Frank didn't wait for the chart. He bolted from his chair and headed for ENT.

"Excuse me, Doctor." It was Maylee's mother. She was leaning over the countertop, hands folded in front of her on the laminated surface.

"Yes, ma'am." I looked up at the woman, dropped my hands to my lap, and rolled forward in the chair. "We'll have her taken care of in no time."

"It's not that, Doctor. I know she'll be fine." She looked down at her hands and shook her head. "I'm just glad this happened and I could get her to the hospital. She doesn't like medical folks—no offense—and won't go see Dr. Jones, our family doctor. But she's got this problem. I'm sure you noticed—it's her weight. She's gained more than a hundred pounds over the past year. I can't be sure, 'cause she won't weigh herself anymore. But she just gets bigger and bigger, and I don't know what to do."

Amy Connors, our unit secretary, glanced at me and then back down at her paperwork.

"Does she have any medical problems or is she on any medication?"

This was a common problem and a common complaint, and always difficult to deal with.

"Well, I think it's all glandular."

Amy cleared her throat and turned a little to one side.

"Glandular," I repeated. "Have you ever tried keeping a log of what she eats? Sometimes that's helpful. Most of us don't realize—"

"She eats like a bird," Maylee's mother interrupted. "I've watched her. We've all watched her. I've seen those TV shows where people sneak candy bars under their clothes. Stuff like that. But she eats like a bird."

"Uh-huh," I murmured, waiting for Amy to clear her throat again and hoping I would be able to maintain my composure. We had heard this story many times.

"It sounds to me like you need to get her in to see Dr. Jones. He might have some ideas about how to—"

"Robert, take a look at this!"

Frank Dixon was hurrying up the hall with a pair of forceps in his hand. He was holding it out in front of him, very much like an Olympic torchbearer. His eyes were focused on the object pinched between the teeth of the stainless-steel instrument.

Maylee's mother spun around, and Amy looked up. Frank reached the counter and held the instrument so that all of us could see.

"It's a…it's a…" Frank was struggling, trying to remember his college entomology.

"It's a candle fly," I casually announced. "And it was in her right ear."

"It's a…How did you know?" Frank sputtered. "It *was* in her right ear. Jeff showed me how to flush it out, and here it is." He raised the deceased insect a little higher.

"That should take care of it." Jeff Ryan walked up behind Frank and laid the chart for ENT on the countertop. "You might want to take a look at this, though." He slid the record toward me. "The vital signs."

"That thing flushed right out." Frank twisted the instrument in his hand, admiring his work. "As soon as I showed it to her, she—" His hand froze in midair and he looked down at me. "How did you know? She didn't say anything about something being in her ear."

"She didn't have to," Amy said, nodding. "It was the dance."

"The dance? What dance?" Frank looked at the secretary, back over his shoulder down the hallway, and finally at me.

"The bug-in-the-ear dance," I solemnly told him. "Usually this time of night. Can't miss it."

"The bug-in-the…" Frank studied the insect again and scratched his head.

I picked up Maylee's chart and held it in front of me.

The vital signs. That's what Jeff had said.

Maylee Strait—27 yr old F. Bug in ear. Heart rate—46. Blood pressure—92/60. Respirations—10. Temperature—96.4.

"Are you sure about these?"

Jeff was looking at me, and he nodded his head. "I repeated them twice, but she looked okay. And she was jumpin' all around with that bug in her ear. I thought we needed to get that taken care of first."

"And her temperature? 96.4?"

"Took that twice too."

"What's the matter?" Frank Dixon turned in my direction, still holding the forceps in the air. "Did I miss something?"

"Come with me." I was up from my chair and around the counter before he could respond.

Maylee was sitting on the stretcher in ENT, leaning back against the wall. Her eyes were closed when we entered the room and slowly opened, but only halfway. She smiled at us again and nodded. Then her eyes closed once more.

"What's the matter?" Frank repeated from behind my right shoulder.

I held up Maylee's clipboard and pointed to her vital signs.

"I didn't take a close—"

"We need to move her into cardiac, Jeff," I interrupted Frank. "Start a line with normal saline and get the lab down here stat. And get a blanket on her."

"Got it." Jeff leaned over, put a hand on the young woman's shoulder, and gently shook her. "Maylee."

Her eyes opened to mere slits again and she mustered a smile, this time more feeble.

"What's going on?" Frank was at her side, helping Jeff get her down on the stretcher. The nurse shrugged and tilted his head in my direction.

"Let's go talk with her mother." I was out the door and hurrying up the hall.

Mrs. Strait was still standing at the nurses' station. She saw her daughter coming up the hall, lying flat on the stretcher and covered by a blanket. Her eyes widened and she clutched her purse to her chest.

She took a step toward Maylee as they wheeled her into cardiac.

I reached over and gently took hold of her elbow.

"Maylee will be fine. We need to start some things and she'll need to come into the hospital. I think you might have been right all along."

She looked up at me, her eyes still wide open. Her mouth was trembling. "What...do you mean?"

"If I'm right, her problem may *be* glandular, in a manner of speaking. All of these signs point to an underactive thyroid gland. Maybe one that's not working at all."

"Her thyroid." Frank Dixon murmured behind me. "That explains her low temperature and heart rate—and her blood pressure."

"That's right." I glanced at Frank and back to Maylee's mother. "As well as her weight gain. How long has she been sleepy like this?"

We talked for a few minutes and it all came together. When her labs returned, the diagnosis was confirmed. Maylee was slipping dangerously close to becoming unresponsive—a coma induced by a nonfunctioning thyroid. If we hadn't caught it and begun aggressive treatment, she would have died.

"I knew something was wrong." Her mother shook her head, tears trailing down her cheeks. "I just couldn't get her to go get help."

Amy leaned over the desk and handed her some Kleenex.

"Thank you." She glanced down at the secretary and something on the countertop caught her eye. Her hand slowly moved toward the forceps Frank had left lying there. She picked it up and held the instrument a few inches from her face.

"Thank the Lord. He used this little bug to save my Maylee's life."

Any Port in a Storm

It started off simply enough, as most conundrums seem to do.

Mildred Jackson brought her eight-year-old boy, Benny, to the ER with chicken pox. That's what she told me it was, and I agreed. He had developed a rash a few days earlier that started on his belly and spread all over his body. He was aggressively scratching the scattered blisters in spite of his mother's strident directives to cease and desist. He didn't have any fever, though, and that was a little odd for chicken pox. I checked his scalp to be sure there were some lesions hidden in his hair—in my experience a prerequisite for the diagnosis. Present and accounted for.

"Well, Mrs. Jackson, I think your boy *does* have chicken pox. Not much to do for it except take some Benadryl for the itching and Tylenol if he develops any fever. Just be sure to follow up with his pediatrician if he has any problems."

She nodded and looked down at her boy. "It's just a little peculiar. I thought he had a mild case when he was two or three. You can't get it again, can you?"

"Not supposed to." I stepped toward the entrance and pulled the curtain aside. "Just be sure to see his pediatrician if there's a problem."

The rash went away, and Benny did fine. Two weeks later, he was back in the ER with the same rash. This time he saw one of my partners.

"Robert, the kid had chicken pox, as sure as I'm standing here."

Jay Barton had seen a lot of kids with the disease and was adamant about his diagnosis.

"But two weeks ago—"

"I know, I know," he interrupted me. "I read your note. And I've never heard of a child getting chicken pox twice, but that has to be what he had. I'm going to check into it and see if this has ever been reported."

We were standing at the nurses' station, and I picked up the chart of the next patient to be seen. Something was bothering me. I looked over at Jay.

"If this *is* recurrent chicken pox, and at his age, he might have some kind of problem with his immune system."

"I thought about that." He put his hand to his chin and slowly stroked the side of his face. "We checked some basic labs, but everything was normal. No low or elevated white count, and his platelets were fine. He looks completely normal, except for that rash."

"Hmm. I'm sure you sent him back to his pediatrician. Maybe he can figure something out. Maybe it will go away again and that will be that."

"Let's hope so." Jay turned and headed toward the medicine room. "Let's hope so."

The rash *did* go away, again. But two weeks later, it came back, just like before. His pediatrician came up to me after a medical staff meeting and told me what had been going on with Benny Jackson.

"Darnedest thing I've ever seen." Jim Matthews was a crusty, cantankerous seventy-year-old curmudgeon, but his patients and their parents loved him. He knew his stuff and didn't waste words or time. "Just like you guys, I thought it was chicken pox the moment I saw him. But three times in a row? That ain't gonna happen. Something else is going on here. He was in the office two weeks after Barton saw him in the ER. Scratching his skin off and making *me* itch. I thought it might be scabies, or some kind of skin mite. But no one in the family has any rash, and they haven't been traveling anywhere. Mildred got a little offended when I mentioned scabies, but I asked her what *she* thought it was and she quieted down. I told her I just didn't know. Never seen anything like it. She told me you boys checked some lab work and I got a copy of all of that. Completely normal. I told her if it didn't go away or if it went away and came back again, we would send him to a dermatologist, or an infectious disease expert."

"How has he done?" This was unusual, and I was really curious about the boy. "Did it go away?"

"Two weeks later, he was clean as a whistle. No bump or blister anywhere. Gone. Haven't seen him since, but it's only been another week or so. I'm just hoping we're through."

"I'm sure Mildred and Benny feel the same way."

But they weren't through. Four days after that meeting, Lori Davidson led Mildred and Benny into the department and down to minor trauma. It was seven in the evening and all of our private rooms were occupied. Mildred shook her head at me as they passed the nurses' station. Benny didn't look up. His eyes were squeezed shut and he was clawing at his trunk and legs.

I picked up the chart of another patient in minor trauma and glanced at the front sheet:

Danny Totherow. 42 yr old M. Bar fight—cut head.

"Looked like he got busted pretty good to me." Amy nodded at the chart in my hand. "Gonna take awhile to put that one back together."

I followed the drops of blood down the hallway and almost ran into Lori when I stepped into minor. She was headed back to triage and handed me Benny Jackson's chart.

"Same thing," she whispered. "He's covered from head to foot."

She slipped around me and disappeared up the hall.

Benny was on the first stretcher on the left, and Lori had pulled a curtain all the way around the bed. Just beyond him, in the back left corner of the room, was Danny Totherow. He was still fifteen feet away, but I could see Amy was right. His scalp was gaping open and still oozing blood. This was going to take awhile.

"How did this happen, Danny?"

I rolled over to him on a stool and looked down at the suture tray Lori had set up. Everything was ready, and I snapped my surgical gloves in place.

Danny was lying on his back, with his bloody head toward the middle of the room. His hands were folded casually across his chest and a smile spread across his face.

"Well, Doc, it was like this." He kept smiling, but didn't open his eyes. His words were garbled and his sentences non-diagrammable, probably the result of cheap wine, the odor of which saturated his breath and permeated the room. From the few words I could make out, it seemed he had been on the losing end of a "broken bottle fight" and was now in need of repair.

"Okay, Danny, I just need you to be still and let me take care of you."

He sighed heavily, nodded his head, and kept smiling.

The curtain behind me suddenly opened, its metal rings shrieking their objection as they were pulled aside.

"Dr. Lesslie, it's me, Mildred Jackson. And Benny."

I slowly spun around on the stool and smiled at her. "Hey, Ms. Jackson. I see Benny has his rash again. Let me take care of this gentleman and I'll be with you as soon as I can. You might want to pull that—"

"You're absolutely right." She shook her head and looked down at Benny. "That rash is back, maybe worse this time. What are we going to do?"

There was no room for an answer. She took a deep breath, puffed it out, and proceeded to present Benny's entire history of the mystery rash. Again.

She didn't leave anything out, from his first visit to the ER up until this latest recurrence. She was especially descriptive of her visits with Dr. Matthews. All the while, Benny sat on the edge of the stretcher, dangling his legs and scratching his torso. I was a captive audience and kept on stitching Danny's scalp.

"You know, my sister in Tennessee wonders if it might be smallpox. But I thought that was a real bad one." She looked down at her son and grabbed his hands. "Stop that, Benny!"

I knew there were a few vials of the virulent smallpox virus locked away in some hidden vault somewhere, but the disease is now nonexistent. Yet it was an intriguing idea. Maybe this was some new and rare malady. One thing for sure: none of us had been able to come up with an answer.

"We've tried everything," Mildred continued from her corner of the room. "Everyone in the house was treated for scabies—I *told* Dr. Matthews—and we washed all of Benny's clothes and sheets. Even steamed them. And now it's back."

I leaned back and reached over to the surgical tray for another piece of suture. Danny Totherow rose up on one elbow and looked over at Benny. A blue surgical towel was draped over his head, but an eyehole allowed him to see the boy. He collapsed back onto the bed and once again folded his hands across his chest.

Benny sat wide-eyed, staring at the apparition across the room. For a brief instant he had stopped scratching. Then he was clawing away again.

"Got a hot tub?"

The muffled question came from under the blue towel.

"What was that?" I picked up an edge of the towel, trying to free his mouth.

"Got a hot tub?"

A lightning bolt had somehow penetrated the building and miraculously struck me. That was the long-sought-for answer.

Mildred Jackson stared at the hooded head of Danny Totherow. "No, we don't have a hot tub. Why?"

Danny mumbled something incoherent, and I took over.

"No hot tub in the neighborhood? No friends or anything with one?"

Mildred shook her head. "No, we don't have one and no one—wait, the Pottses have one in their backyard, Charlie's one of Benny's friends. But he's not allowed to get in it. That's the only one I know of. Why?"

"Uh-huh," came the slurred response from Danny.

"Benny, you haven't been in Charlie's hot tub, have you?" Mildred was staring at her son and he dropped his head, shaking it slowly.

"Benny?" She dragged his name out, hanging it in the air.

With eloquent fluidity, just as a master conductor would direct his orchestra, Benny's head-shaking morphed into a slow but definite nod.

"I'm sorry, Momma. Charlie said it would be okay, and his mother didn't mind, as long as I didn't have the rash when I got in."

"Has Charlie ever gotten this rash, Benny?" I had turned around on the stool, my gloved hands upright in front of me.

"No, he never did. He never got in the tub. Said it was too dirty."

"Uh-huh." Danny again.

That was it—the answer—the resolution of our mystery. *Hot tub dermatitis,* usually caused by the pseudomonas bacterium. Its small blisters look very much like the lesions of chicken pox. The Pottses' tub was a regular petri dish—and every time Benny's rash cleared, he would dip himself in it again.

I explained all this to Mildred Jackson.

"Well, I'll be. And that's it?"

"That's it. We shouldn't be seeing him again with this rash."

Case closed.

I spun around again and looked down at Danny Totherow's covered head.

My seafaring grandfather's words came back to me: *Any port in a storm.*

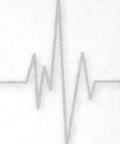

The Cell Phone

"Sharon, what is it going to take to get through to you? How many times do I have to tell you about picking up hitchhikers?"

Mike Brothers had just walked into the house and was hanging up his jacket. His wife, Sharon, was standing in front of the kitchen sink, preparing chicken for the frying skillet.

She froze and stared out the window. *How had he known? Who told him?*

"Mike, I don't know what—"

"No point in denying it. That guy you picked up in the rain out on Highway 5 yesterday used to work with the rescue squad over in Union. He was at the station this afternoon when I went by to pick up some paperwork and told me what happened. He said to thank you again."

"See." Sharon turned around and dried her hands on her bright-orange apron, which was emblazoned with a bold Clemson Tiger paw. "That *was* the right thing to do. It was raining and he was in the middle of nowhere with his car broken down. He needed a ride. What was I supposed to do?"

"Call someone—anyone. Call 9-1-1 and let them deal with it. Just don't stop and pick up a stranger. Again, *I* knew the guy, but *you* didn't. It's just not safe anymore—not these days."

Sharon turned back to her chicken. "Okay, I hear you. I'll try not to do that again."

"Sharon…"

"Alright, I *won't* do that again."

Mike shook his head and headed to the den.

Sharon and Mike Brothers were paramedics and worked as a team on EMS 1. In his "off time," Mike did heating-and-air work with his uncle.

Once a month their supplier, Charlie Stokes, would drive from Columbia in his pickup truck, carrying parts and equipment the two men had ordered.

Over the years, Charlie had almost become a member of the family. If Sharon was off duty and knew he was coming, he would find a plate of oatmeal cookies on the kitchen counter, still warm from the oven, and freshly made iced tea.

"Nobody makes tea like you do, Sharon."

"I'm going to tell your wife you said that, Charlie," she warned one afternoon.

"Go ahead. She knows. And by the way, tell me about that three-wheeler out in the shed."

Mike had bought the recreational vehicle years ago when their son was young enough to be interested in it and not girls. He was in college now, and the unused three-wheeler was languishing under the lean-to of Mike's shop behind the house, covered by a camo tarp.

"You interested?" she asked him. "I'm sure Mike would be glad to sell it—probably not for very much, if anything. He might just *give* it to you."

"Does it still run?" The last cookie disappeared from the plate and Charlie wiped some renegade crumbs from his mouth.

"You know Mike. Of course it runs."

On his next monthly visit, Charlie came prepared to load the over-sized bike into his truck. Mike refused to accept any money for it and helped his friend lift it into the back of the pickup. They couldn't get the tailgate closed and had to strap it securely to whatever hooks and handles they could find.

Satisfied, Mike stepped into the shed and came back with a roll of yellow tape imprinted with large black letters.

Crime Scene—Do Not Cross

"We keep a roll of this on the unit *just in case*." Mike tore off several five-foot lengths of tape and tied them to the three-wheeler. "This should satisfy the Highway Patrol."

"I'm gonna be going slow," Charlie said, checking the straps one more time. "Only have one more delivery to make, out on Beckley Church Road. Then I'm headed home. My ten-year-old is gonna be excited when he sees this. Thanks, you two."

Sharon and Mike stood in the driveway and watched Charlie Stokes turn onto the highway. He waved one last time through his open window, and then was gone.

Two hours later, Mike's radio flashed and beeped from the kitchen table. They weren't on duty, but he usually kept it on in case they might be needed.

A dispatcher's strained voice reported a gunshot wound off Highway 5, their part of the county.

Sharon looked at her husband. "Do you think we—"

"Police on the scene," the dispatcher continued. "And the coroner is en route. EMS not required."

Mike shook his head. "They won't need us for this one."

Later, they were getting ready for bed and Sharon switched the TV on to a Charlotte station. A reporter was standing with his microphone, silently mouthing his report.

Mike was the first to see the scrawl on the bottom of the picture and shouted, "Turn up the sound! Quick!"

"...on Beckley Church Road. Police officers say they have a suspect in custody but have released no other details about his identity. They won't yet release the identity of the victim, who was found facedown in a ditch beside the road with two bullet wounds—one in the back and one in the head."

The reporter was not at the scene of the shooting but was standing in front of police headquarters, downtown. The cameraman slowly scanned away from the reporter, pointing his lens toward a cordoned-off area of the parking lot.

"We are told that the suspect was stopped while driving this vehicle and was subdued after a brief struggle."

The camera zoomed in on a blue pickup truck. The view shifted as the cameraman walked behind the vehicle. Shadows played over the back of the truck and the camera shook until he finally came to a stop. The truck's tailgate was down. Yellow ribbons of tape fluttered limply in the night breeze, tied to the back of a three-wheeler.

Mike and Sharon stared at each other.

The reporter's voice cut into the heartbroken silence of their bedroom. "It appears the driver of this truck may have stopped, picked up the suspect to give him a ride, and was then shot and killed."

Mike flipped off the TV.

After Charlie Stokes had been killed by a hitchhiker, Mike didn't have to say anything more to Sharon. She watched her husband grieve the death of his friend and knew what was in his heart and in his thoughts. She didn't want to add to his sadness.

Months passed, and it was the dead of winter. Mike and his uncle were out on a call to a failing heat pump and freezing family, and Sharon was returning home from the grocery store.

"Well, I'll be."

It had been cold and overcast, but no one had called for snow. She switched on the windshield wipers, clearing some stubborn flakes clinging to the tempered glass. The inside of the SUV was warm and toasty, but she cranked up the heater a notch—just for good measure.

The snow was coming down harder, and Sharon squinted to see the road ahead, driving in the middle of the highway and not the right lane.

"What in the world…"

There was something up ahead, something on the side of the road.

She slowed, sped up the windshield wipers, and stared into the late-afternoon gloaming.

Just ahead, walking on the right shoulder of the road, was the figure of a man. He was hunched over, hands thrust deep in the pockets of his pants, with a short-sleeved shirt on.

"What in the world…"

Sharon was barely crawling as she drew alongside. The man looked at her, chin tucked to his chest, and forged forward into the blowing snow. His face—the man was probably in his late twenties—was pink and chapped.

She hesitated, but only for an instant. The SUV accelerated and she headed home, only moments away.

Sharon jumped from the running vehicle, ran inside without her groceries, and stood staring in front of the coatrack in the laundry room.

"Which one…"

She grabbed an old hunting jacket of Mike's—its sleeves worn and tattered—hurried back to the car, and tossed it onto the passenger seat. Over the faded camo on the back was taped a large, orange "X"—one arm of which was missing.

"This should work." Sharon patted the jacket, shifted into reverse, and headed back to Highway 5.

What if he's gone? What if someone picked him up? What if something worse has...

She cleared a curve in the road and there he was, huddled against the snow and wind, persistently plodding forward.

Sharon slowed as she approached the man and kept the SUV in the middle of the road. She came to a stop beside him and he once again looked up at her. This time he didn't continue walking, but stopped and turned to face her. His lips were blue and ice was dangling from his scruffy beard.

That poor man is freezing. I've just got to give him a ride.

She looked to her right and reached for the hunting jacket.

Her cell phone started to hum and vibrate on the console. She picked it up and glanced at the caller ID. It was Mike. She stared at the phone, and with each vibration she heard another of Mike's warnings. It vibrated one last time, and she saw the face of Charlie Stokes.

Sharon dropped the cell phone to her lap, grabbed the coat, and twisted around in her seat. The hiker stood shivering just outside her window, his hands still buried in his pockets. She hit the button for the window and lowered it just enough to be able to push the jacket into the arms of the surprised young man.

"Here, I hope this helps. I'll call someone to get you a ride."

She raised the window, sprinted a hundred yards down the road, whipped around in a deftly executed U-turn, and headed back to her home.

The man was clumsily getting into the jacket as she passed.

"Why didn't you answer my call?" Mike had just walked into the kitchen and dropped his hat and gloves on the table.

"I couldn't get to it in time," Sharon answered, mostly in truth. "Was it something important? I figured if it was, you'd call back."

"Nope. Just checking on you."

Mike turned on the small TV set on the counter and sat down.

"Boy, it's cold out there," he said. "Freezing."

They both heard "Highway 5 in York County" and jerked around together, staring at the television.

Mike turned up the volume and they moved closer to the screen.

"This comes after the monthlong investigation of multiple home invasions in western York County. Twenty-nine-year-old PJ Bartlett was arrested this evening while walking down Highway 5 in an unexpected snowstorm. He has been charged with multiple counts of forceful breaking and entering, grand larceny, and malicious vandalism. He is in York at the County Detention Center with no possibility of bail. When arrested, he had two knives and a small-caliber handgun in his possession."

Mike shook his head. "I saw some police lights on my way home, but I had no idea."

He tensed and leaned closer to the television, his forehead almost touching the screen.

Walking between two stout officers, his back to the camera, was the suspect. He was wearing a faded camo hunting jacket with a large, orange "X" on the back. One arm of the X was missing.

"Hey, isn't that my jacket?"

Sharon stepped back from the television, pale and trembling. She put her hand on the table to steady herself and it came to rest on something.

She looked down, picked it up, and clutched it to her chest.

Her cell phone.

The *Miracle* of a Changed Heart

I will give you a new heart
and put a new spirit in you;
I will remove from you your heart of stone
and give you a heart of flesh.
and I will put my Spirit in you…

Ezekiel 36:26-27

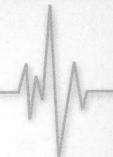

A Demon

"You know that guy?"

I looked up at the police officer standing at my side at the nurses' station. He nodded down the hallway behind me.

"Him. That guy going into minor trauma."

I turned just in time to see the profile of a slender, hunched-over man disappearing through the doorway. It was enough.

"Yes, I've seen him here in the ER before. Why?"

I looked down at the chart on the countertop and resumed making a few notes. For a moment I struggled for the man's name, but gave up. I knew he had emphysema, smoked like a freight train, but I couldn't remember his name. Probably a sad commentary—remembering people by their diseases and not by their names.

"That's Jasper Reynolds."

The name sounded a little familiar, but I had work to do. "Hmm." I didn't look up.

"He was one bad actor."

"Was?" I looked over at the officer, now curious about Mr. Reynolds—who seemed to be very much in the present.

"Oh yeah. You know about the 'Friendship Nine' problem we had here in Rock Hill? Happened back in the early '60s."

That sounded familiar, and I remembered hearing something about it. But I didn't know much more than it involved the civil rights movement. I glanced up at the officer and studied his face. He wasn't old enough to remember anything from the '80s, much less the '60s.

"Apparently it wasn't Rock Hill's most shining moment." He leaned an elbow on the countertop and tapped his pen on the notepad in front of him. "Some of the older guys on the force used to talk about it. It was a sit-in at one of the diners downtown, with students from Friendship

College—that's why they call it the 'Friendship Nine'—and it ended with all of them being arrested."

He looked down at the notepad, his pen now making lazy, looping circles.

"What does that have to do with Jasper Reynolds?"

"Chief Jones told me that Jasper was a troublemaker, and caused a lot of problems during that incident. Caused a lot of problems after that too. He was high up in the Klan, I think. Got into a lot of trouble in the '60s and '70s. If there was a rally going on or something being burned down, you could bet that Jasper was in on it.

"I know when I first came to town and started on the job, I arrested him a couple of times for disorderly conduct and inciting stuff. Always had some friends with him, never by himself it seemed. A gang, you could call it. He's a small guy, can't weigh more than a hundred and fifty, but they warned me he was quite a brawler. I know the first time I picked him up, he gave me all I could handle. After that, I would always call for backup. Like I said, he was mean."

There was that past tense again. I glanced down the empty hallway to the doorway of minor trauma. Hard to imagine that the slumped-over, wheezing, and chronically short-of-breath Jasper Reynolds I knew could have such an infamous past. That's what the officer must have meant. Jasper wasn't much of a brawler anymore. He had a hard time just making it down our hall without having to stop and rest.

"Here's the chart for minor trauma C." Amy Connors slid the clipboard across the countertop. "The triage nurse thinks his wrist is broken, so I've filled out an X-ray request."

"Thanks." I picked up the chart and scanned the patient ID information. *Darnell Reynolds. 6 yr old male. Fell and injured right wrist.*

Reynolds. Must be related to Jasper—maybe his grandson.

"See ya later, Doc." The officer scooped up his notepad, tipped his hat to me and then to Amy, and turned and walked out of the department.

I was halfway to minor when James Green, one of our orderlies, turned the corner in the back hallway and headed straight toward me. He was humming a familiar tune—a hymn, I thought. James was in his early sixties and had been working at the hospital since finishing high school. His father had been an AME minister, and James had been singing in the church's gospel group since he was able to hold a hymnbook.

"Hey, Dr. Lesslie." His ever-present and infectious smile spread across his face and he almost skipped as he came up the hall. As he passed the doorway to minor trauma, he glanced into the room. And suddenly stopped, frozen where he stood. His mouth dropped and his fists clenched. I stopped and watched, never having seen him act like this before.

Finally, he took a deep breath, turned up the hallway again, and took slow, ponderous steps toward me.

He was still trembling, his smile replaced by an angry scowl.

"You know who that is back there, Doc?" He jerked his head behind him. "That's...Jasper Reynolds."

The name hung in the air, dripping with disgust and loathing. What had gotten into this gentle man?

"He and a bunch of his friends burned my family out of our house. Daddy had scars on his arms from pulling us kids out before the fire got us. I haven't seen him in years and years, but that's him, I know it. That man is just plain evil."

I didn't know what to say, and just stood there. James's head slumped to his chest and his shoulders gradually relaxed. He slowly nodded his head, then began mumbling something I could barely make out. "I know it's wrong to feel this way, to let that man get to me like this. I know it's wrong."

The moment passed, and James stood up straight. His smile hadn't returned, but the scowl was gone.

"Got work to do, Doc. Got work to do."

He stepped around me and walked up the hallway to the nurses' station.

I glanced down at the chart in my hands. Jasper Reynolds. What manner of demon awaited me in minor trauma? My jaw tightened and my heart quickened, hardened first by what the young police officer had told me and then by James Green's tragic story.

Bed C, in the back right corner, was the only occupied stretcher in the room. Jasper Reynolds was sitting on it. His scrawny legs dangled over the edge and his body was turned away from me, one arm draped over a little boy. I could see the child's sneakered feet, but that was all.

"Papa, it hurts real bad," the boy quietly sobbed.

"It's gonna be okay, Darnell. We're gonna get you fixed up." Jasper's voice was raspy from decades of smoking.

I walked across the room and the man looked up. "Hey, Doc, not me this time." He managed an awkward smile and coughed twice. "It's my grandson here. I think he broke his arm."

Keeping one arm firmly around the boy's shoulder, he turned and shifted a little on the stretcher. I saw Darnell leaning heavily into Jasper's chest, and I froze, my feet anchored in the middle of the room.

The animosity I felt for this man disappeared, washed away in an instant.

It was obvious that Jasper loved this boy.

And the boy—Darnell looked up at his grandfather with large, trusting eyes. His hair, lustrous black with tight curls, brushed his grandpa's sleeve. And his skin was a dark, rich shade of brown.

"Papa?" the little boy said quietly.

"It's okay, Darnell. Dr. Lesslie is gonna take care of you."

I walked over to the stretcher and sat down beside Jasper Reynolds.

This man was no longer a demon.

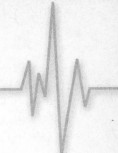

Joy to the World

"I love you, Dr. Rob."

The last stitch was in place and I was dabbing some stray drops of blood from the twenty-year-old's right eyebrow.

"I love you too, Manny."

Manny was lying on a stretcher in minor trauma, smiling up at me with the innocent, loving face of a child with Down syndrome. He and his mother were regulars at our church's Just Joy service.

She walked over beside me and put a hand on her boy's shoulder.

"We're going to have to be more careful when there's ice on the sidewalk, aren't we, son?"

Mid-January had gifted us with a late-night storm of ice and freezing rain, blanketing roads and sidewalks with a slippery sheet of shiny glass. Manny had bolted out the front of his house, down, down the steps, and into a lamppost. He was lucky he had only injured his eyebrow.

"Listen to your momma, Manny." I stood up and stretched. "We'll see you in a week to take these stitches out."

Lori Davidson pulled the curtain closed behind me, filling the last of the four minor trauma beds.

"Have a seat on the stretcher, Mr. Conyers. One of the doctors will be with you in a few minutes."

She was looking down, making a note on the man's chart, and we almost collided in the doorway.

"Oh, excuse me." She stepped back and adjusted her reading glasses.

"Here, let me take that." I reached for the clipboard in her hand.

"Eighty-two year old gentleman," she said quietly. "Another ice injury. Slipped on his front steps and fell. Looks like he's broken his wrist."

I glanced at the stretcher to my right. Jim Conyers slouched on the bed, cradling a crudely splinted left wrist. It appeared he had rolled a copy of an old *National Geographic* around his forearm, then wrapped it with duct tape. Clever.

He looked up at me as I stepped over, his eyes scrunched up with pain.

Something behind me captured his attention and he leaned to one side, peering around me. His face broke into a wide grin and his eyes beamed.

With his good hand, he reached into a shirt pocket and took out a wrapped piece of peppermint candy. His eyebrows arched as he stretched out his hand. "Is it okay, ma'am?"

I turned around to find Manny and his mother standing behind me. His eyes were wide and his head bobbed up and down.

His mother looked at her son and then Mr. Conyers. "Sure. That's fine."

Manny sprang over to the man and happily took the piece of candy.

"What do you tell the nice gentleman?" she reminded him.

"Thank you." Manny's eyes were focused on the treasure in his hand. He struggled for a moment and finally managed to remove the wrapper. He popped the red-striped mint into his mouth. "Thank you."

The bear hug startled me and I gasped for breath. Manny had walked up to the nurses' station and grabbed me from behind.

"Let go of Dr. Rob." His mother quickly stepped over and put a gentle hand on his shoulder.

He was strong, and the release was immediate. I twisted around and looked again into the smiling face of the young man. He nodded and stepped back a little.

"Wait just a minute." I reached out and grabbed him. "I think I need another one of those hugs."

He squeezed me again, with every bit of his heart and body and soul. When Manny hugs you, you know you've been hugged.

He could have stayed like that all day, but his mother said, "It's time to go, son."

"Just be careful out there, Manny," I told him. "And don't do any more ice-skating."

He waved at everyone in the department as he and his mother disappeared through the triage door.

I heard the quiet, distinctive chuckle of Harriet Gray and spun around to face the grandmotherly nurse. She had been watching all of this from the other side of the counter.

"You know who that is, don't you?" She folded her arms across her chest and rocked from side to side.

I glanced behind me at the triage entrance. "Manny?"

"No, the elderly man back in minor. The one on the stretcher *beside* Manny."

I shook my head, confused.

Harriet smiled and nodded. "That's Jim Conyers. Let me tell you about him."

Jim and Gertrude Conyers had lived in a large antebellum house on Main Street, back when it *was* the main street. They had never had children of their own, and "adopted" those in the surrounding neighborhoods. "Aunt Gertie" always had fresh-baked cookies in her kitchen, and "Uncle Jim" would show the kids his long rows of muscadine vines in the backyard and let them take as many of the grapes as they could carry. Each Christmas, they could be counted on to have "a little something" for any child that happened to knock on their door. And there were a lot of knocks.

All that changed when Gertrude was diagnosed with cancer. She died slowly, and her last months were painful. The brightly lit house on the corner of Main Street darkened, as did Jim Conyers. He became sullen, withdrawn.

"He wasn't mean or anything," Harriet added quietly. "He just wasn't… He wasn't Uncle Jim anymore." She paused and shook her head.

"Every year, our church choir goes Christmas caroling. We'd always stop at Jim Conyers' house, somebody would knock on the door, and we'd sing a couple of songs. He never came out—never opened his door. One year he even turned off the porch lights while we were singing. Then a few years ago, my teenage granddaughters went caroling with me. They brought a friend, and that friend's little brother had tagged along. He couldn't have been more than six or seven, but he knew the words to all the songs and wasn't shy about singing out. Not always in key, mind you. But he was having a grand time.

"It was getting late, about nine o'clock, and we found ourselves in front of Jim Conyers' place. Somebody knocked on the door and we stood in the front yard and sang two or three songs. Nothing. The door never opened, but we could see him moving around inside.

"We turned around to head to the next house, and I'll never forget what happened. We had started singing 'Joy to the World' and were almost to the street when my granddaughter's friend realized her little brother was missing. She ran through the crowd, looking for him, calling out his name, but he wasn't there. Then someone hollered out, 'Look! Up on the porch!'

"We turned around and that child was standing all alone on Jim Conyers' porch. He was knocking on the door, quiet as a lamb, but absolutely determined. He never stopped. We all sort of froze, and then his sister took off—but it was too late. The door opened and out stepped Jim Conyers himself. He glowered at us and didn't move a muscle. I don't know if the boy said something or moved a little, but Jim looked down at his face and just stared. All of a sudden, that boy reached out and grabbed Jim's legs and just held on.

"Jim looked over at us and then at the boy. No one said a word. No one dared to. Finally, Jim's hand slowly came up, and he put it on the boy's head."

Harriet stopped, her eyes moist and distant.

"And then?"

She cleared her throat and looked at me. "That was it. He patted the child's head a couple of times and the boy let loose of his leg, turned around, and bounced down the steps. It wasn't till he got out to where we were standing, under the streetlight, that I saw."

"Saw what?" I was leaning on the counter now, not wanting to miss a single word.

"That child had the sweetest face—all smiles and happiness and love. He had Down syndrome, just like Manny."

We stood there for a moment, looking at each other, and for an instant were removed from the chaos of the ER—we were somewhere else.

"What about Jim Conyers? Did he come out on his porch the next time you went caroling?"

"Oh no." She chuckled again. "He never comes out and stands on his porch. He always meets us in the front yard with a plate of cookies."

I glanced down the hallway, to the doorway of minor trauma.

"I need to go talk with this Jim Conyers." His clipboard was still in my hand. I stood up straight and turned in his direction.

Harriet stopped me. "It's Uncle Jim."

Let every heart prepare him room.

The *Miracle* of Faith

*Now faith is confidence in what we hope for
and assurance about what we do not see.*

HEBREWS 11:1

*Faith is the bird that feels the light
and sings when the dawn is still dark.*

RABINDRANATH TAGORE (1861–1941)

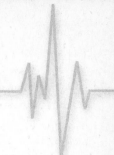

Blessed Assurance

"Yeah, Doc, right there. That's where it hurts."

My hand was pressing lightly into the pit of Clay Winston's abdomen, just below the lower end of his sternum. I didn't feel any masses or anything unusual. But this seemed to where his gnawing pain was originating.

Clay was a close friend of Harriet Gray, and she was waiting for me at the nurses' station when I walked out of room 4.

"Well, what do you think, Dr. Lesslie?"

I dropped his chart onto the counter and scanned his vital signs again. No fever and normal blood pressure and pulse. His weight seemed a little low—162 pounds—and I circled it with my pen. He was six feet tall and might normally be slender, but I had no point of reference. I had never—

"He's been losing weight." Harriet tapped his chart with her index finger, right where I had just circled it. "I've never seen him this skinny, and he looks pale. What do you think's going on?"

I scratched my head, trying to put all of this together. My first thought had been his gallbladder. He had been having intermittent belly pain for the past few weeks, usually brought on by eating. And there was always the possibility of reflux or even an ulcer. But the weight-loss thing bothered me. That opened up a whole different set of possibilities.

"I'm not sure, Harriet. We need to check some things while he's here— some lab work and maybe an ultrasound. And I agree, he *does* look a little pale. We need to find out what's causing all this."

"I've known him since high school." She glanced over at the curtained entrance of room 4. "He's a great guy. I just hope he's alright."

Clay Winston was not "alright." His lab work came back with elevated liver enzymes and evidence of a chronic anemia. But that wasn't his real worry.

"Dr. Lesslie, this is Dr. Newton over in radiology." Amy reached over the countertop and handed her phone to me. "He wants to talk to you about the ultrasound in room 4."

I still had Clay's lab slips in my hand, and dropped them before grabbing the receiver. A sudden uneasiness crept over me. It was unusual for the radiologist to call about an ultrasound report. Ordinarily we just got a faxed piece of paper with their impression scribbled on it.

"Bryan, this is Robert. What have you got there?"

"Hi, Robert. Listen, this Clay Winston, with the gallbladder ultrasound." There was a pause, and my uneasiness grew. "His gallbladder is fine—no stones or signs of infection. But there's something going on in his pancreas." Another pause, and I waited. "There's a mass in the head of the pancreas, and it looks like cancer. If that fits with what you're seeing, we'll need to get a CT scan."

It *did* fit. I thanked him, handed the phone to Amy, and asked her to arrange for a CT of Clay's abdomen. Then I walked over to room 4.

I pulled the curtain aside, and Harriet looked over at me. She and Clay had been laughing about something—both were still smiling. My eyes met the nurse's and the smile froze on her face.

"Mr. Winston, we need to talk about your ultrasound and your lab work."

I pulled up a stool and told him what we had found and what needed to be done. When I said the words "pancreatic cancer," his eyes closed, but only for an instant. He looked over at Harriet and nodded.

"I knew something was wrong, and something more than just my gallbladder. But pancreatic cancer...Isn't that a bad one, Dr. Lesslie?"

It *was* a bad one, and we talked about it. If it indeed was pancreatic cancer, the chances of his being alive a year from now were very small.

Clay accepted all of this with the same calm demeanor he had exhibited when he first arrived in the ER. He nodded a lot, and occasionally pursed his lips. But he was calm, almost resolved.

The curtain was drawn aside and Amy Connors stuck her head in the room.

"They're ready for Mr. Winston in CT."

A few minutes later, his stretcher disappeared around the corner in the back of the department. Harriet pulled me aside. "He's only sixty years old and has always been healthy. I just don't understand how something like this can happen. Especially to someone like Clay. He's one of the kindest people I've ever known—always there if you need him." She stopped and looked down at the tiled floor. "I know it happens to all of us. It's just that…This is going to be hard."

The next six months *were* hard for Clay. The diagnosis of pancreatic cancer had been confirmed, and he had been to several leading cancer centers. The answer was always the same—there was nothing anyone could do. It was only a matter of time.

And time was running out. We saw him in the ER every few weeks, and on each visit he was paler, more emaciated. We were watching him pass from this life.

Yet his attitude, his spirit, remained undaunted. In spite of his pain, he was able to smile, ask about the staff members he had come to know, and apologize for "being a bother."

On one of his final visits, I overheard Harriet talking with Lori Davidson in the medicine room.

"We go to the same church, you know," the older woman was saying. "And everyone who knows Clay has been praying for him. But you know what he said last week? He told my husband and me that the Lord had already answered his prayers."

I was standing just outside the room, eavesdropping. But I felt no guilt. I didn't want to interrupt these two women. And I did want to hear what Harriet was saying.

"He told us he had always prayed for the Lord's help to live his life well, and that now he was praying for the strength to die well. And that his prayer was being answered."

Clay Winston *was* dying well. The last time I saw him alive was on a Tuesday morning in the middle of December. His skin was parchmentlike, his eyes sunken but still sparkling, still calm. And he still smiled.

"How does that happen?" Jeff Ryan whispered. We were standing at the nurses' station, talking about Clay and whether we should try to have him admitted to the hospital. He was close to the end, and a better option would be to keep him in the ER for several hours, with people who knew and cared for him. That might be all the time he had left.

"You mean his attitude?" I turned and looked into Jeff's eyes. Like the rest of us, he had come to know and respect Clay.

"Yeah, how does that happen?"

I looked past him to room 2, then put a hand on his shoulder. "Come on—let *him* tell you how this happens."

We walked over to room 2, drew aside the curtain, and sat down beside Clay's stretcher. He was awake and looked up as we entered.

"Gentlemen, I didn't press the call button by mistake, did I?"

"No, we just wanted to talk a minute, if you feel up to it."

His breathing was labored, but when I explained why we were in the room, he looked over at Jeff. His face suddenly brightened and his eyes began to dance.

"Jeff, this is the easy part. My battle is almost over, and I'm not facing it alone. I'm sure of that. That assurance means everything. You see, it comes down to faith, and that's a gift from the Lord. When you experience the real presence of the Lord in your life, that faith becomes something else—something stronger, something rock solid. I would call it assurance. Blessed assurance."

Clay glanced over at me and nodded.

He took a couple of deep breaths, turned back to Jeff, and smiled.

"That's how it happens."

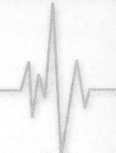

I Have a Plan

"How many stitches, Doc?"

I had just numbed up Jeremy Draffin's lacerated eyebrow and hadn't started putting it back together yet. This was a frequent question with patients and I understood his concern, but I had no clue—and wouldn't until we were finished.

There are a couple of ways to answer this. If my patient has been imbibing or is under the influence of some other mind-altering substance, I will sometimes answer, "Somewhere between fifty and sixty." That usually evokes an interesting response, at which point I give them my best estimate. Jeremy was completely sober and had suffered this injury while practicing basketball at one of the local high schools. A friend's elbow had been in the wrong place at the wrong time. I decided to give him my best estimate.

"Probably seven or eight. We'll count them when we're finished."

His mother was standing on the other side of the stretcher, and I knew the next question.

"Will there be a bad scar?" she asked.

"It's impossible to cut the skin without a scar," I answered—which is true. "But this is mostly in his eyebrow and should pretty much disappear." Which is also true. "I think in a couple of months he'll forget it happened." True once again.

"I hope so," she cooed. "He's such a handsome young man."

Twenty minutes later, I was standing at the nurses' station, putting the final notes on the teenager's chart. The wound had come together perfectly and would in fact disappear in a few months. Lori was leading mother and son up the hall and Mrs. Draffin stopped beside me.

"Thank you, Dr. Lesslie."

I turned and said, "He should do fine. Remember, the stitches need to come out in six or seven days."

Over her left shoulder I watched as her son used his mother's makeup compact to examine his eyebrow. Gingerly he touched the skin around it, tilted his head at multiple angles, then flicked the unruly locks of hair on his forehead back into place.

"I just hope this doesn't scar," he mumbled.

Jeff Ryan rushed through the triage door. "Got a bleeder here, Doc."

Behind him followed an ashen-faced middle-aged man—Charlie Stilman.

"Trauma 3 is open." Lori gently but firmly moved the teenager out of the way and Jeff and his patient moved quickly down the hallway. Charlie caught my eye and gave me a weak smile. I looked down at his bandaged and bloody hand and my heart thumped in my chest. It was his *left* hand—his violin-fingering hand.

Charlie Stilman was in his early fifties, and we sang together in our church choir. He was an accomplished violinist, often lending his musical gift to our worship services. Though classically trained, he frequently swapped his violin for a fiddle and played with a local bluegrass band.

Drops of blood followed Charlie and Jeff as they disappeared into minor trauma.

"Watch out, Jeremy. Don't step in that." Behind me Mrs. Draffin was pointing to the tiled floor and the scattered splashes of crimson. She grabbed her son's elbow and followed Lori out through the exit.

Charlie was lying on bed C, in the back-right corner of the room. Jeff was standing beside the stretcher, carefully unwrapping the makeshift bandage—what appeared to be a blue-gingham kitchen towel.

"A fine mess here, Robert." Charlie's color was better and he almost looked relaxed with his uninjured hand behind his head. He looked up at Jeff. "Do I need to raise it higher? Is this okay?"

"You're doing fine, Mr. Stilman." Jeff reached for a handful of gauze and prepared to remove the last of the towel. He dropped it to the floor— a thin stream of blood arched a foot into the air. The nurse quickly pressed the gauze over the torn vessel and held it tightly.

"You're right," I said, moving over to Jeff's side. "He *does* have a bleeder."

"I did a good job, didn't I?" Charlie was looking at his wounded hand.

In that brief glimpse, I had seen enough to know we had a real problem. His index, long, and ring fingers were filleted, with torn tendons exposed and dangling.

"How did this happen, Charlie?" I walked around him to the storage cabinet and grabbed a pair of sterile gloves.

"Jimmy and I were in the shop working on some bluebird houses, and I guess his hand…my hand slipped and got pulled into the table saw. It happened in the blink of an eye—that quick. I've always been careful, but—"

"Is Jimmy okay?" I doubted he had been injured physically. It was his emotional state I was worried about. Jimmy was Charlie's sixteen-year-old son, and the two were very close. If he was somehow responsible for this, it would be difficult for him.

Charlie looked up at me and studied my eyes. I raised my eyebrows and waited. He smiled, nodded, and said, "I'll make sure he's okay."

We got the pain under control and I was able to get a good look at Charlie's torn and ripped-up fingers. It was worse than I had thought. There were a couple of obvious fractures and of course the lacerated tendons, but the blood supply to the fingers was intact.

"The good news, Charlie, is that you're not going to lose anything. The bad news is—"

"The bad news is my fingers will never work the same again. I knew that the moment it happened."

I was studying his injured hand and didn't say anything. When I finally looked up into my friend's face, he was smiling.

"I know. You're thinking about my violin. Or maybe my fiddle—I think you always preferred me playing that instrument. Well, those days are over."

I was trying to imagine the intricate fingering of the fretless violin, the delicate touch required to make it sing. And I knew Charlie was right. Those days were over.

"Robert, which of the Bible prophets do some people call the 'whining prophet'?"

"What?" *Where had that come from? We needed to talk about his hand and what the next steps would be. Yet here was a Bible trivia question.*

I thought for a moment and ventured, "Jonah, I suppose."

"Good thought, but not correct. It's Jeremiah. A lot of people just think of him as a whiner and unfortunately don't spend much time studying what he has to say. He *does* do a lot of whining, I suppose, but he was dealing with some tough times, and bad things were about to happen. But some of my favorite passages in Scripture come from his writings.

"One of those came to mind as Jimmy drove me over here. I know you're familiar with it. It comes from the twenty-ninth chapter—not sure which verses. I can't quote it exactly, but it has to do with the Lord having a plan for us—a plan for something good. I thought if Jeremiah could say that with the Babylonians breathing down Israel's neck, who was I to complain about a table-saw blade? I know he has something planned for me, something good." He paused and raised his wounded hand a few inches from the arm board. "This is just a detour, and a small one at that. Like you said, I'm not going to lose anything. But even if I did, it wouldn't matter—not really."

Jimmy walked into the room and over to his father's side. "Are you going to be alright, Dad?" He glanced down at the gauze-covered hand and quickly looked away.

"I'm going to be fine, son." He reached out and took his boy's hand in his good one. "We'll both be fine."

Six months passed. Charlie had been singing in the choir, his hand slowly healing from three separate surgeries. His thumb was fine, as was his little finger. But the other digits were stiff, useless. One Sunday morning he didn't join us in the choir room before the worship service. *Odd.* I had seen him earlier and knew he was at the church.

We filed into the choir loft without him and our organist nodded, signaling for us to sit. Then he looked to his right, over the curtain behind him, and nodded again.

I could see heads turning in the congregation, necks straining, eyes searching.

The sanctuary was silent, and I heard soft footsteps approaching the raised platform and podium. Then a head came into view, then an upper body.

It was Charlie Stilman. He stopped just behind the organist and nodded. His eye caught mine. He smiled and gave me a wink.

The organist began his prelude, something majestic and triumphant. After a few measures, Charlie took a deep breath and raised a bright, shining trombone to his lips. He began playing, and the sanctuary was filled with the mellow, rich tones of the instrument, expertly played.

How had he learned to play this in only a brief six months?

His right hand deftly and gracefully handled the slide, while the only requirement for his left hand was to steady the instrument.

It was beautiful and amazing.

As the last blended notes of the organ and trombone faded into the far reaches of the sanctuary, one lone, vibrant voice from the back of the church uttered what was in all our hearts.

"Amen."

"I know the plans I have for you,"
declares the LORD,
"plans to prosper you and not to harm you,
plans to give you hope and a future."

JEREMIAH 29:11

Outside Looking In

How many times had I seen the two of them walking up the hill of the ER parking lot? How many times holding hands, slowly getting into that '82 Oldsmobile station wagon and driving off?

"It's different now, isn't it?"

Virginia Granger startled me, and I turned to face the head nurse. I was standing in the medicine room, gazing out the window as Ed Reynolds disappeared into the inky midnight blackness of the ER parking lot. Alone.

"Yeah," I sighed. "It's different."

"He seems okay." Virginia moved beside me and stood hands on hips, looking out the large window. "But he's what? Almost ninety? They were together a lot of years."

"He's ninety-two." Lori Davidson walked into the room and dropped the clipboard of the cardiac room on the counter. "That's what he just told me. Julia was ninety, and they were married sixty-five years."

"Sixty-five years," Virginia quietly repeated. "It *is* going to be different now."

——

"Make yourself comfortable now, Mr. Reynolds. This is going to take awhile."

I had first met Ed Reynolds twenty years earlier when he came to the ER with a Skilsaw laceration of his left hand. Actually there were three separate lacerations of his fingers and palm. He was lucky—there was no tendon or bone injury.

"I've always wondered why they call it a '*skill*' saw," he chuckled. "If I had any skill, I wouldn't be in this fix."

Ed and I hit it off from the very beginning. He was my father's age and seemed to have the same outlook on a lot of things. Maybe it was a generational thing. Maybe it was their shared experiences as veterans of the Second World War that drew me to him.

We talked continuously while I put his hand back together. Initially it was about the weather and sports—nothing very deep. He liked the Dallas Cowboys and I liked the Washington Redskins, and I threatened to not use any more lidocaine if he needed something else for the pain. He asked where I was from, and about my parents. When I told him about my father and about his college career being interrupted by the war, Ed grew quiet. He didn't say anything for a few minutes, and I focused on his shredded index finger.

"We landed in Normandy," he said quietly. "There were six of us, close friends. And we fought together all the way into Belgium. It was during the Battle of the Bulge that...everything changed. They say it was the bloodiest American battle of the war. All I know is that only two of us survived the fighting." He grew quiet again, and his head slumped on his chest.

Julia had been sitting on a chair near the door. She got up, stepped over to her husband, and put a hand on his shoulder.

Ed sighed and raised his head. "That's where I got my medal." He patted his right thigh with his good hand. "A piece of shrapnel from a tank shell almost took my leg off. Still have it in there somewhere—wouldn't let them take it out. When the weather changes, or it gets cold, it starts to hurt. And I remember."

"Tell him the rest, Ed." Julia was grinning now, and she patted his shoulder.

"Oh yeah. Like I said, this is my medal." He was laughing now, and slapping his thigh again. "But I usually spell it with a 'T.'"

I shook my head. "Mr. Reynolds, that's pretty bad."

Later, as he was walking up the hallway, I noticed his limp.

"It gets worse when he's tired." Julia was walking beside me and nodded at her husband. She put a hand on my elbow and we stopped. "Dr. Lesslie, Ed doesn't talk about the war. You should feel honored."

I glanced at Ed Reynolds and then at his tall, slender wife. "I *am* honored. I'm glad I got to meet him, and you."

The following Easter, Ed was in the ER again. This time it was because of weakness and shortness of breath when he walked for any significant distance. I was worried it might be his heart, and we would have been happier with that diagnosis. It turned out that his weakness was due to chronic blood loss from colon cancer.

"Well, we'll just have to deal with it." He reached out, took his wife's hand, and they looked at each other. There was fear in her eyes, but not Ed's. He nodded and smiled at her. "We're going to be alright." Then he looked at me and said, "What's the next step, Dr. Lesslie?"

He *was* alright after his surgery. The tumor was completely removed and he never had any recurrence or any other problem with the cancer. But there were other things awaiting Julia and Ed Reynolds. They were passing from their seventies into their eighties, and their bodies were beginning to fail. One early winter, Julia contracted the flu, which was complicated by pneumonia. In her weakened condition, she tripped one night, fell, and broke her hip.

I was worried, and I told Ed so. At her age, with pneumonia and now a fractured hip, there was a significant chance she wouldn't survive.

"I'm afraid the odds aren't in her favor," I told him.

He nodded slowly and his brow furrowed, but only for an instant.

"Whatever happens, Dr. Lesslie, she'll be fine. *We'll* be fine. We'll hope for the best, but you know that the best is something beyond all of this." He waved his hand expansively around him. "Julia knows that. She's in the Lord's hands. We're *both* in the Lord's hands."

Julia's hip was operated on, and she defied the odds. Every day she grew stronger, and miraculously she was able to go to rehab and then home.

For three or four years we didn't see either of them in the ER. I ran into Ed a couple of times in town, and on one of those occasions he told me about his heart disease.

"Nothing serious yet." He was grinning, and his large paw of a hand gripped my shoulder. "No surgery or anything like that. The cardiologist just has me on a couple of medications. Julia, though, is a different story. She's had to have three stents put in. We've been lucky that she hasn't had a heart attack—caught it in time. But she can't get around like she used to."

In the end, it was a heart attack that had brought her to the ER this final time. Julia had collapsed at home, and when the paramedics arrived she barely had a pulse. She made it to the hospital, but with Ed standing by her side, holding her hand, she breathed her last.

―――

Lori reached into her jacket pocket and took out a worn, yellowed piece of paper.

"Ed Reynolds gave this to me, just before we left the cardiac room."

She opened the folded note and carefully spread it out on the counter, smoothing the creases and crimped corners.

"He said he wanted us to have this. It was Julia's, and he said she didn't need it anymore." She looked up at us, her brow furrowed, and she shook her head. "And then he said something about her being on the right side of the door."

Virginia adjusted her bifocals and we crowded together over the neatly handwritten note.

At present we are on the outside of the world,
the wrong side of the door.
We discern the freshness and purity of morning,
but they do not make us fresh and pure.
We cannot mingle with the splendours we see.
But all the leaves of the New Testament are rustling
with the rumor that it will not always be so.
Someday, God willing, we shall get in.

C.S. LEWIS,
from *The Weight of Glory*

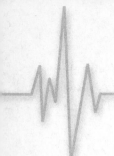

Lila

Samuel Jefferson's heart had stopped fifteen minutes ago. Lori Davidson had turned off the cardiac monitor and quietly walked out of cardiac, leaving me with the fifty-eight-year-old's wife, children, uncle, and mother.

I was standing against a far wall, wanting them to have this time together and ready for any questions they might have—if there were any I could answer.

Samuel's death had not been a surprise. Six months earlier he had been diagnosed with an aggressive brain tumor and his course had been rapidly downhill.

"He must have bled into the tumor," I had told them. "From that moment he was completely unconscious."

I don't know if they had heard me, or if it made any difference. But he hadn't suffered, not today. That part was over.

His wife stood by the stretcher, flanked by their son and daughter. They held each other and cried.

At the head of the bed was Lila, Samuel's mother. She stood statue-like, resting her hand gently on her son's shoulder. Her eyes were moist, but there was a smile on her face. Every few seconds, she silently nodded.

Ed Jefferson, Samuel's uncle, walked over beside me, his footsteps amazingly quiet for such a big man.

He leaned close and whispered in my ear. "I know it was expected—we all knew it was a matter of days. But it's still...It's hard." He nodded his head in Lila's direction. "This is the third child she'll bury. I can't imagine...You're just not supposed to bury your children."

Three children. How could that be? How could this frail eighty-year-old deal with that kind of loss?

"She must be a remarkable woman," I said quietly. "I don't know how she can remain so peaceful and calm."

"And strong," Ed added. "She's the glue that holds this family together. And I don't know either. I think it must have started when Gordon died—her husband. He was my brother."

He motioned toward the doorway and I followed him into the hall.

———

Ten years earlier. Gordon and Lila Jefferson lived fifteen miles outside town on a two-hundred-acre farm. Their three boys had grown up, gone off to school, and settled elsewhere.

The land had been in the family for over two hundred years and had successfully supported several generations with cattle, cotton, and soybeans. Gordon had decided to try his hand at growing apples and planted five acres of several different varieties. It was among those newly budding trees that he had his heart attack.

Lila knew something was wrong. Gordon was late coming in for dinner—unusual for him—but it was more than that. She just *felt* something was wrong and went out looking for him.

She found him—propped up against a tree—pale, sweating, and short of breath.

"Sorry, honey. I tried to get back to the house, but I couldn't make it."

It was a bumpy ride in the ambulance—through the apple trees, down some rutted tractor paths, and across a rolling cow pasture—but he was still alive when they reached the hospital. The ER doctor quickly diagnosed a massive heart attack and arranged for an immediate heart cath.

Lila was waiting in the family room with two of their sons. There was a knock on the door and Gordon's cardiologist stepped into the crowded room.

"Your husband is stable...for the moment. A large part of his heart muscle is dead. He had two vessels that were almost completely blocked and we were able to place stents in them. That should help. But his heart is very weak, and he's not a candidate for bypass surgery. We're going to move him upstairs to the CCU and watch him closely."

Samuel stood up and rubbed his hands together. "You said he's stable for *now*. What does that mean?"

"I'm afraid it means that your father is a very sick man, and there's a good chance...There's a good chance he won't survive this."

Samuel stared at the doctor, then looked down at his mother. Her face was tired, worn—suddenly years older.

"I'd like to see him," Lila said, stumbling to one side as she stood up.

Samuel reached out and steadied her.

"We'll be getting him upstairs as soon as—"

"I'd like to see my husband." She stood up straight, pulled back her shoulders, and stepped toward the door. No one was going to stop her.

She left her two sons in the family room and followed the cardiologist to the cath lab. Gordon was lying on a stretcher in a small holding area. IVs were inserted in both arms and hands, and an oxygen mask covered his mouth and nose. Cardiac monitor leads dangled snakelike from the edge of the thin mattress.

Lila moved carefully around the equipment and stood beside her husband, gently laying a hand on his damp forehead.

His eyes opened to drowsy slits and he smiled at her.

"Who's going to get the cows in?" he chuckled weakly.

Lila didn't smile. She studied her husband's face, noting every line and crease and wrinkle. "What am I going to do with you, Gordon?"

One of the cath lab nurses walked up behind Lila and lightly placed a hand on her shoulder. "Ma'am, we're almost ready to move him to the CCU. You'll need to step out into the hallway."

Gordon nodded and raised his left hand. Lila grasped it and shook her head. "What am I going to do with you?"

He pulled her close and said, "Lila, listen...I—"

"You'll be out of here in no time." She squeezed his hand and squinted at him. "You'll be calling those cows in and—"

"Lila, that's not going to happen. Just remember that I love you—I always have—and I'll be okay. You will too."

She opened her mouth but no words escaped.

"Ma'am," the nurse quietly spoke again. "You'll need to step outside."

In a few moments she was alone in the hallway, staring at the ceiling and taking long, sighing breaths. Her troubled, tired mind wandered through dark and threatening rooms—rooms she had always been too afraid to unlock—and she closed her eyes.

The air above her exploded.

"Code Blue! Cath lab!" the overhead intercom blasted. "Code Blue! Cath lab!"

Lila's frail body jerked and she stumbled backward, almost falling.

She stood frozen in the hall—wide-eyed—mouth gaping. A set of footsteps—then two, three—came pounding toward her. She moved against the far wall as a team of hospital staff members descended on the cath lab. Through the closed door she heard orders being barked, metal carts moving and clanging, excited shouting. Minutes passed, and then... silence.

It was Gordon. He was gone.

She stood in the hallway, her eyes closed now, waiting.

Gordon's cardiologist stepped through the door and stood before her. He was flushed and sweating. His eyes moved to the floor and he slowly began to shake his head.

"Mrs. Jefferson, I'm afraid—"

She raised her arms over her head and started running. She didn't know where she was going, and she didn't care. In her mind she was screaming, but no sound passed her lips.

It was midnight, and a corridor stretched empty in front of her. She reached its end and stumbled left, past the closed doors of sleeping patients. Then a right, aimlessly following this unfamiliar and impersonal labyrinth.

"Lila."

The voice came from behind her—unfamiliar. She ran on, shaking her head.

She turned another corner, this time into a shorter corridor that ended abruptly in a large, uncurtained window.

"Lila."

The voice again, just behind her.

She reached the end of the hallway and her weathered, work-hardened palms slammed into the plate glass. There was nowhere to turn, nowhere to hide.

She gasped for breath and her hands fell to her side.

With slow, shuffling steps, she turned around.

The hall was empty.

She took another deep breath and shook her head.

"Lila."

The voice was behind her again. She spun around, her face inches from the window, and stared into a black, cloudless sky. A sliver of moon was off to her right, and just above it was a star—bright and shimmering, larger than she had ever seen. It was billions of miles away but looked so close…

"Lila."

She searched the dark sky…her eyes returned to that singular star. The voice was coming from somewhere in the night, no longer unfamiliar. It surrounded her, and the sound of her name warmed and calmed her.

"Lila, he is with *me.*"

She knelt in front of the window, her hands outstretched on the cold tile floor. And she cried.

~~~

"I don't think she's cried since that night, when Gordon died." Ed slowly stroked his chin and looked into my eyes. "She's had plenty reason to, with her other two boys. Lee was killed in an auto accident and James had a heart attack. It was hard for her, of course. But she was the strong one in the family—just like now. She's the rock."

The door of cardiac opened and Lila Jefferson stepped out. She saw the two of us and walked over.

"Thank you for what you did, Dr. Lesslie." She smiled at me, then turned to Ed.

Lila took his giant hands and cradled them in her own.

"Ed, I've always known where Samuel's heart was, and I *know* where he is now. I know where they *all* are."

I am the resurrection, and the life:
he that believeth in me, though he were dead,
yet shall he live:
And whosoever liveth and believeth in me
shall never die.

Jesus, in John 11:25-26 (KJV)

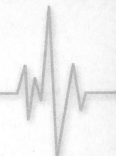

A Benediction

David Youngblood was taking a shortcut on his way home from Greenville and was making good time on India Hook Road. He passed Bonnybrook on his right, made the next turn in the road, and slammed on his brakes. Traffic was backed up as far as he could see and was barely moving.

Must be an accident up ahead.

He settled back in his seat and glanced at his watch. Ten-fifteen a.m. He still had plenty of time to make it to the neighborhood cookout.

Minutes dragged, and he crawled with the other cars toward Celanese Road, where things should clear out. Ahead, near the Westminster school, he saw the flashing lights of police and emergency vehicles.

Twenty minutes passed, and he was near the cluster of patrol cars and ambulances. Policemen, firemen, and paramedics were standing in groups talking, and one lone officer was waving the line of traffic forward. Whatever had happened was over now. David glanced toward his left to the side of an EMS unit. A bike lay crumpled in a heap in the tangle of tall grass.

I was hot and sweaty, and it took an effort to pull my golf bag out of the car's backseat and hoist it to my shoulder. My wife and I were at the beach for a few days, and I had just finished a round of golf with a friend.

"Let's get cleaned up and see what our brides want to do."

"You mean her?" He pointed to a third-floor balcony where my wife stood waving her arms and calling my name.

I couldn't understand what she was yelling, but something was wrong. I hurried to the elevator, pushed the "3" button, and waited.

The door slowly opened. Barbara was standing in front of me. Her face was drained of color and her lips quivered.

What was wrong? The kids? My father? Her parents?

"I've already packed our things." Her voice trembled and she shook her head. "We've got to go—now."

I stood staring at her, jumbled thoughts twisting through my mind.

"Barbara, what—"

"John is dead."

I shook my head. I didn't grasp what she'd just said, I must have…

"John is dead."

The four-hour trip to Rock Hill was a blur. Without cell phones, we were cut off from family and friends, left with only a few scant pieces of information to try to piece together. All we knew for sure was that the world had been turned upside down, changed forever.

John was the thirteen-year-old son of two of our closest friends, Walter and Jeanie, and one of the best friends of our two sons, Robbie and Jeffrey. Somehow, he was dead. But maybe—just maybe—that was a mistake.

We drove straight to Walter and Jeanie's home, and the truth was right in front of us. They lived in the back of a cul-de-sac, and it was filled with cars and people. I turned in, hoping to find a place to park.

"Stop and let me out." Barbara reached for the door handle and I had barely come to a halt before she was gone, hurrying toward the house.

Cars were pulled onto neighbors' lawns, and every conceivable place to park was occupied. I slowly made my way to a nearby street, found a spot, and began to jog back to the house.

"Hey, Robert."

I stopped in the middle of the road and turned around. David Young-blood, a good friend of mine, was hurrying to catch up.

"I'm glad you're here," he said, puffing.

We shook hands and I nodded.

We walked in silence—my mind spinning, chasing tangled threads of thought.

"I saw his bike."

My head jerked toward him.

"Out on India Hook. Some crazy driver swerved off the road and…he died instantly."

The vision played itself out in my mind and I shivered in the muggy June heat.

We turned into the cul-de-sac. People were everywhere, milling around the yard, whispering, shaking their heads. They would silently nod when we made eye contact.

A group of teenage boys was standing under a basketball goal at the end of the driveway—heads down, hands stuffed in pockets.

David's head turned in their direction. "It's really going to be tough on all his friends."

My boys! And my daughters! I have to find them!

"My kids—" I waved a hand toward David and hurried up to the front door. I was barely able to squeeze into the foyer when I walked in. A quiet murmuring filled the house and I glanced around, trying to find Barbara.

Jeffrey, our younger son, had been at the beach that week with Walter's sister, brother-in-law, and their children. I searched the dining and living rooms but couldn't find him.

Audrey, David's wife, tapped my shoulder. "Barbara's upstairs with Walter and Jeanie."

I made my way to the bottom of the stairway and took two or three steps. My hand was on the rail, and I stopped—empty and drained. A huge weight pressed down on me. I couldn't begin to know the pain and devastation Walter and Jeanie were experiencing. Just the very thought—

"Daddy!"

I turned toward the front door and saw Jeffrey standing there, looking up at me.

He slipped through the crowd at the bottom of the stairs and bolted up to where I stood waiting.

Our eyes met. No words were spoken. We wrapped our arms around each other...and cried.

We stood that way until Audrey came to the bottom of the steps. She nodded to me, reached out, and took Jeffrey's hand.

"Let's go find Robbie and your sisters."

I needed to find them too. But first I needed to see Walter and Jeanie. "Your mom and I will be down in just a minute, Jeff." I turned and walked heavily up the stairs.

I tapped lightly, opened the door, and stepped into our friends' bedroom. Walter was pacing in front of the far window. Jeanie was sitting beside Barbara on the bed, and the two had their arms around each other. The door closed quietly behind me.

A cloud descended over Rock Hill and over and around the people who knew and loved John and his family. Even strangers—or those whose lives barely had been touched by this family—sensed that something was different. Something was lost. We were lost.

The next few days were a blur—dragging painfully into a future none of us would have chosen.

We settled into an uncomfortable but necessary routine. Family and friends would make their way to Walter and Jeanie's home. Children and teenagers would gather, trying to find comfort and security with each other—each of us seeking our way through this sorrow.

Yet in the midst of this darkness there were welcomed glimpses of light. Whether it was with friends at church, my coworkers in the ER, or our children and their friends, the conversations always turned to John:

"What about that time at church camp when we decided to take our bikes down that steep hill in front of the hotel at Bonclarken? Everybody chickened out except John. When he finally made it back to the dining hall, he was all scratched up and bleeding—and he was grinning from ear to ear."

"You remember when some older kids were picking on McAuley? John was a head shorter than they were, but he stood right in front of the meanest one and backed him down. And then the whole bunch high-tailed it outta there. I'm tellin' ya, he was the man."

"I've never met a boy who could make people laugh like John. He would walk in a room with those blue eyes twinkling and people couldn't help but start smiling. There was just something special about his spirit."

"Momma told me about a time right after Christmas. Uncle Walter was at work and Aunt Jeanie had to go out of town. She'd told John to start taking down the decorations while she was gone, and Momma went over to check on him. When she got there, he was flying around the house on his Rollerblades, cramming stuff into a big black plastic bag. She said she would've yanked a knot in him if she coulda caught him."

"Now that sounds like John."

"What about the time..."

Moments of light. But always—always—the cloud.

A few weeks later, several of us were sitting with Walter and Jeanie in their living room. Bright sunshine filtered through the large windows, sharply contrasting with the somber mood within. Pictures of John were everywhere—on the mantel, tables, bookshelves. Maybe they had always been there and I was only noticing them now.

Jeanie sat beside her husband on the sofa. Her hand absently stroked a small glass frame—with a picture of John in a baseball uniform.

The conversation was strained, trivial. Walter nodded from time to time, but Jeanie was miles—worlds—away.

Someone asked her a question, but she didn't answer. She looked down at the picture for a few moments, and a small smile started to appear on her face. She paused a moment longer, then set the frame on a nearby table.

"Listen, there is something I want to share with you all." She folded her hands and leaned forward a bit. "It happened a day or so after John's accident."

Her eyes were brightening and her smile grew. A palpable energy began to fill the room.

"Just before the funeral, the four of us went to see John. We were still in shock, we still couldn't believe it had all happened. One of the attendants at the funeral home showed us into the little room where John's...casket was resting. I remember the man saying, 'Stay as long as you need.' And I'm thinking, *What I need is my son back.*"

Walter moved closer to his wife and gently laid a hand on her forearm.

"At first we just stood around him, all quiet. Walter and I tried to be strong for our girls. But how could we?" Her voice broke a little. "I prayed for some message of hope and reassurance for them—something undeniable, some small sign." She looked down at her teacup on the table. "But I knew it wasn't just for them. Walter and I needed it just as much."

She paused and looked into her husband's reddened eyes, reached over, and squeezed his hand.

"I was standing at the casket, looking down at him...at my son. He was dressed in his favorite saxophone shirt and blue-jean shorts. Then I looked down at his left wrist, and there was his watch, somehow still running after the accident. I didn't know why, but it struck me as amazing, really remarkable. I began to stroke his hair, and I thought how normal it felt...how alive." She stopped for a second, and took a sip of tea. "Then...

then I touched his skin. It was cold. And the reality of his death came crashing in once more."

Tears were streaming down Jeanie's cheeks now, but somehow she was still smiling. *How was she able to tell us this and find the strength to hold it together?* I bowed my head and rubbed the tears from my own eyes.

"We all held each other and we cried and cried. I silently prayed again for the Lord to give his peace to us…to put his arms around us…to let us know he was with us. My heart was, well, shattered, and I felt so terribly empty. I had no more words—nothing. But just at that moment, I found myself turning to Walter and the girls and saying, 'The Lord *is* with us, and he wants us to know that.'

"And right then—*beep-beep…beep-beep-beep*! It was the alarm on John's watch. It cut through the silence. We all looked at each other—we were stunned, just stunned. There's no other word to describe it.

"And then we were able to smile at each other, even through our tears. In his love and kindness, the Lord had spoken to us. He was holding John—and his Holy Spirit was holding us."

I was stunned, and I watched as Walter put his arm around his wife. There was a powerful, peaceful hush in the room, and Jeanie leaned back in the sofa.

"And he's *still* holding us."

Two months later, the family traveled to Amelia Island. They needed to get away—relax—spend time together, alone. They had never been to this beach, and there would be no painful memories. Walter and Jeanie wanted it to be as "normal" as possible, if anything could ever be normal again.

It was a long trip from Rock Hill, and they collapsed into their beds soon after arriving. The next morning, Walter and Jeanie woke the sleepy girls and led them down the walkway to the beach. The tide was out, and the deserted sand stretched before them.

"I want us to see the sunrise," Walter told his family. On the dark eastern horizon, a purplish light was rising, growing. Minutes passed, and the purple changed to red, then orange, and the glow gradually flooded the beach around them. This was God's gift to his creation each morning—his promise of a new day, a new beginning.

"Look!"

Every eye was drawn to the sand at their feet. At first no one spoke, stunned by what they thought they were seeing. The light grew brighter and there was no longer any question. They laughed and cried and hugged each other.

Written in six-foot-high letters was the name

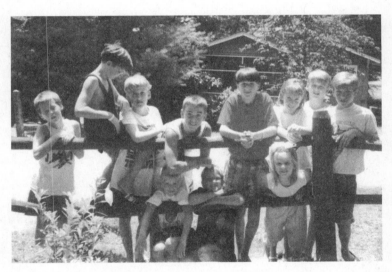

Hunt, Jeff, Walt, John, Robbie, Maria, Vance, Brian
Dixon, McAuley, Elle

With humble thanks to Walter, Jeanie, Letty, and Maria—
and with eternal praise to God the Holy Spirit,
their Comforter and Friend.
Amen and amen.

—✳—

Miracles are a retelling in small letters
of the very same story
which is written across the whole world
in letters too large for some of us to see.

C.S. Lewis (1898–1963)

—✳—

About the Author

D<small>R</small>. R<small>OBERT</small> L<small>ESSLIE</small>, bestselling author of *Angels in the ER, Angels on the Night Shift, Notes from a Doctor's Pocket,* and *Angels on Call, Angels and Heroes,* is a physician who lives and actively practices medicine in Rock Hill, South Carolina. Board-certified in both emergency medicine and occupational medicine, he is the co-owner of two busy urgent care/occupational clinics.

For more than 25 years, Dr. Lesslie worked in and directed several of the busiest ERs in the Charlotte, North Carolina, area. He also served as medical director of the emergency department at Rock Hill General Hospital for almost 15 years. During his tenure as medical director, he received the American Medical Association's Continuing Education Award. He also traveled around the country, giving lively, innovative lectures to the Emergency Nurses Association at their annual meetings in major cities.

For seven years, Dr. Lesslie wrote a weekly medical column for *The Charlotte Observer* presenting a wide variety of topics, both medical and editorial. He also pens a regular column on medical, philosophical, and personal topics for the *YC,* a monthly publication in York County, North Carolina.

Dr. Lesslie enjoys the fast-paced environment of the ER and the need to make rapid and accurate diagnoses. He views his medical career as an opportunity to go beyond simply diagnosing and treating individual patients. For him, it is a way to fulfill a higher calling by meeting the real physical and emotional needs of his patients.

An active member of his home church in Rock Hill, Dr. Lesslie serves as an elder, and he and his wife, Barbara, teach Sunday school and sing in the church choir. They are also involved with an outreach program for disabled/handicapped individuals, Camp Joy, where Dr. Lesslie serves as the camp physician for a week each summer. He also enjoys mentoring high-school and college students considering a career in medicine.

Dr. Lesslie and his wife, Barbara, have been married for more than 35 years. Together they have raised four children—Lori, Amy, Robbie, and Jeffrey—and are now enjoying five grandchildren. In his spare time, Dr. Lesslie enjoys gardening, golf, hunting, reading, and bagpiping.

www.robertlesslie.com

Also by Robert Lesslie, MD

Notes from a Doctor's Pocket
Heartwarming Stories of Hope and Healing

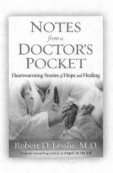

These *Notes from a Doctor's Pocket* come from the decades of experiences of bestselling author Dr. Robert Lesslie. Here you'll meet up with the characters, coincidences, and complications that surround the life of an ER doc:

- characters like Freddy, who literally shoots himself in the foot
- coincidences such as finally having the chance to hear what patients say to each other when doctors and nurses aren't in the room
- complications like the hospital nurse's feud with her sister and how they find forgiveness

These heart-tugging, heart-lifting slices of life will prompt you too to search for opportunities to give the comfort of a touch, the grace of a kind word, or a prayer that brings hope and healing.

Angels on Call
Inspiring True Stories from the ER

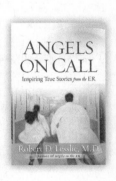

Dr. Robert Lesslie shares experiences—some heartwarming, some edge-of-your-seat—that reveal answers to those often unspoken pleas of "Who can I turn to?" "Who's on call for me?"

> …Sally Carlton and Wanda Bennett are both in desperate situations. But sometimes the passion for life burns where least expected.

> …Wesley Wood is rushed through the doors on a stretcher, undergoing CPR from a 300-pound nursing attendant sitting on his chest. He clearly needs some help—but how?

Throughout these remarkable accounts, you'll also catch glimpses of those who are now asking, "Who am I on call *for?*" It is these people who have found the kind of healing we all need.

Angels and Heroes
True Stories from the Front Line

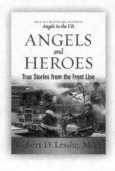

Every day, courageous men and women from the police, fire, and EMS face danger with the grace and strength of angels. Dr. Robert Lesslie gives you a new appreciation of their amazing experiences as he takes you close-up to...

- breathtaking moments from the front lines of the police
- heart-pounding incidents with firemen
- poignant accounts from the men and women of EMS
- and unforgettable heart-and-soul rescues from the ER

In these remarkable true stories you'll see the human connections and the divine moments of the heroes among us...and be encouraged to watch for those times when you too might be able to rescue someone with God's love and care.

Angels on the Night Shift
Inspirational True Stories from the ER

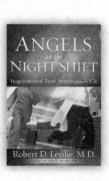

During the darkest hours of the night—and our lives—we need someone to comfort us and help us endure. Sometimes a nurse, a doctor, another patient, even a stranger is the "angel" who sees us through till the sun rises again.

In these remarkable glimpses into the heart of the ER, Dr. Robert Lesslie opens the curtain on the fears, hopes, conflicts, and resolutions that go on even as illnesses are treated, lives are saved, and griefs are dealt with. You will gain a window on some of life's greatest wonders and mysteries while you share the joys and struggles, the failures and redemptions, of people just like you.

More Inspiring Reading from Harvest House

Glimpses of Heaven

Surprising Stories of Hope and Encouragement

Bestselling authors Kay Warren, Gordon MacDonald, Liz Curtis Higgs, Mark Buchanan, Virginia Stem Owens, and Ben Patterson are among the 50 contributors to this collection of brief, inspiring stories. The goodness of God, the value of every person, and the importance of meaningful relationships are just a few of the glimpses of heaven you'll experience through these first-person accounts:

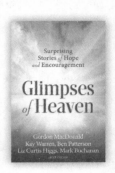

- Kay Warren spontaneously joins a welcome-home celebration for soldiers at an airport and witnesses the power of encouragement.

- Gordon MacDonald helps a friend struggle through a long hike and discovers the meaning of true friendship.

- Liz Curtis Higgs befriends a young fellow passenger but learns something from him about her "baggage."

You'll love these engaging stories and will be inspired to see how your own day-to-day life is brimming with significance...when you choose to view it through the eyes of faith.

Four Paws from Heaven

Devotions for Dog Lovers

M.R. Wells, Kris Young, and Connie Fleishauer

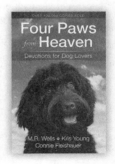

Friend, family member, guardian, comforter—a dog can add so much to our lives. These furry, four-footed creatures truly are wonderful gifts from a loving Creator to bring joy, laughter, and warmth to our hearts and homes. These delightful devotions will make you smile and perhaps grow a little misty as you enjoy true stories of how God watches over and provides for us even as we care for our canine companions.

Dogs to the Rescue
Inspirational Stories of Four-Footed Heroes
M.R. Wells

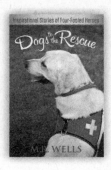

From the beloved author of *Four Paws from Heaven* (nearly 125,000 copies sold) comes a new devotional for everyone who's ever loved a dog. This collection of short devotions features inspirational stories of rescue dogs, therapy dogs, and dogs that help their humans in unexpected ways. Discover

- what pets can teach us about the love of the Master
- the blessings of obedience
- how helping a friend can help you too

These heartwarming tales of doggie heroics will teach you that who you are on the inside matters most—and that with God (and a furry friend!) on your side, there's no obstacle you can't overcome.

Heavenly Cat Tales
Devotions for Those Who Love Them
M.R. Wells, Connie Fleishauer, and Dottie Adams

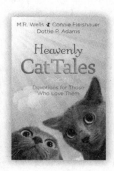

For those with the right cat-itude, there is nothing like a nice kitty to make life great. Cat people love cats not because they are purr-fect, but in spite of their flaws. These entertaining and enlightening devotions will delight you as you discover how God daily draws us to Himself, provides for our every need, and loves us purr-fectly in spite of our flaws.